Arise, And Fly Free!

A Holy Spirit-Led Guide to Healing for Post-Abortive African American Women.

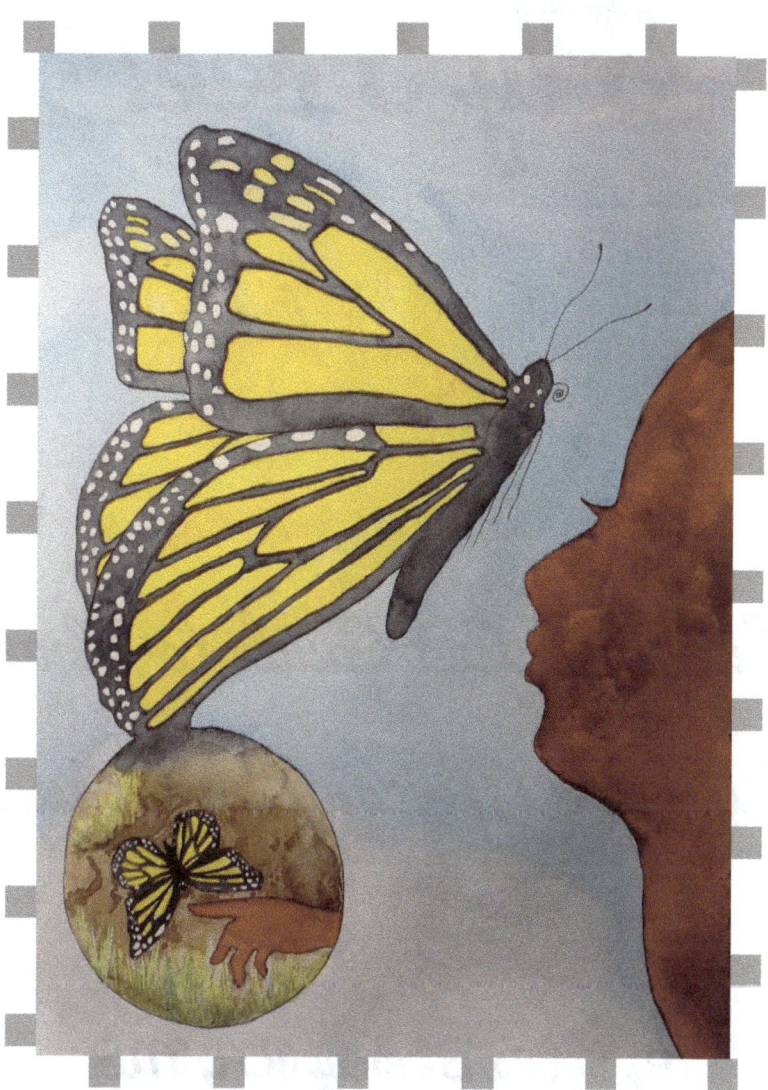

By Sylvia Blakely RN, MS,
Founder, Arise Daughter and Arise Artists

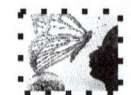

Arise, And Fly Free!

A Holy Spirit-Led Guide to Healing for Post-Abortive African American Women

By Sylvia Blakely RN, MS

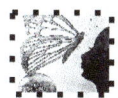

Arise, and Fly Free: A Holy Spirit-led Guide to Healing for Post-Abortive African American Women
Publishing Consultant: Lakeya Tucker, www.mltconsulting.net
Copyright © 2024 by Sylvia Blakely. All Rights Reserved.
First Edition, November 2024
ISBN No. 979-8-218-55351-7

Unless otherwise noted, all Scripture quotations are taken from the Holy Bible, New Living Translation (NLT).

All material in this book is protected by copyright under U.S. copyright laws and is the property of Sylvia Blakely. You may not copy, reproduce, distribute, publish, display, modify, scan, create derivative works, alter, transmit, exploit in any way, sell or offer for sale any of the content produced in this book over any network without the author's permission. For permission to use the content in this book, please contact arisedaughter@gmail.com

Please be aware that the nature of this book is dynamic and that the hyperlinks, though working at the time of publication, could break or otherwise become corrupted in the future. The fact that a link may no longer work should not alter your enthusiasm for searching out the material by title. Please note that the eBook complements this print version, and it may be used simultaneity to interact with the links.

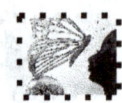

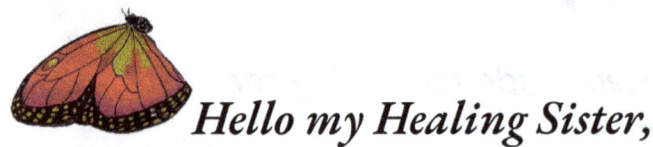 *Hello my Healing Sister,*

This book is solely the property of our almighty God. Please share this study with others whom you know have been stuck in the muck for WAY too long! Our heavenly Father loves us so much that He wants us healed, whole and free. Our King Jesus came to minister, suffer, die and rise again because He loves us too much for us to stay stuck in sin and our Comforter, Holy Spirit, loves us way too much to allow us to do life without Him.

   Share your healing, share this book and together, let's shame the devil!

So Christ has truly set us free. Now make sure that you stay free, and don't get tied up again in slavery to the law.
Galatians 5:1 NLT

Sylvia Blakely, RN, MS.
Founder: AriseDaughter.org and AriseArtists.com

The Mission of Arise Daughter:
We are post-abortion mentoring ministries equipped by Holy Spirit to help women and men heal, train and serve in the Kingdom of God.

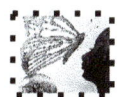

ACKNOWLEDGEMENTS

I want to start by thanking my heavenly Father for the 'download' that happened in the wee hours of an extremely cold January morning in Washington, D.C. If it had not been for Him, this book would not have been conceived nor written.

I also want to thank my husband Raymond for steadfastly standing next to me no matter what the Lord calls me to do for Arise Daughter and Arise Artists.

A hearty "thank you" goes out to Chandra White-Cummings who listened to my idea, looked at my handwritten outline and said, "Sis, you've got something here!" Her enthusiasm gave me the push to start.

Thank you to my bestie and book illustrator Freda Abbott Ayodele for the beautifully hand drawn book cover and to my cousin Roxanne Fields for our unforgettable Arise Daughter logo. I love you both to life!

A very special "thank you" to early book reviewers: Freda Abbott-Ayodele, Annette Crouch, and Karen Jenkins. Your love and commitment to God and healing His children is palpable.

This book would not be coherent if not for the editorial support of Ms. Britani Anthony, Dr. Anita P. Jackson, Ms. Karen Jenkins, and Ms. Chandra White-Cummings. Thank you all for making me a better writer.

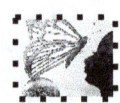

Final chapter reviews were completed as 1:1 studies with: Freda Abbott-Ayodele, Veronica Davis-King, Annette Crouch, Karen Jenkins, Sharon Fordham, Roxanne Fields, Raymond Blakely, and Schearice Moore. You shared your heart, your time, and your invaluable comments and for that I am grateful.

Last but certainly not least, I'd like to thank my Arise Daughter and Arise Artists sisters whose healing journeys inspired my writing.

*Note that you will find links to titles used as reference materials throughout the curriculum. Feel free to read what interests you at your own pace. The books and articles are informational only and the views are not necessarily endorsed. This is a healing curriculum and not a work of rigorous scholarship-please treat it as such.

Disclaimer and TRIGGER ALERT: The material in this book may trigger unresolved feelings surrounding your abortion(s) or other past trauma so please, read with caution. The online resources referenced in the chapters are not meant to be substitutes for licensed mental health professionals. Neither the author nor contributors are counselors or therapists; we offer peer to peer support only. Feel free to consult with a licensed therapist or counselor as needed either before, during or after going through the material in this book. The Suicide Prevention number is 988 which you can text or call. H3Helpline.org is a 24/7 resource for post-abortive women and men.

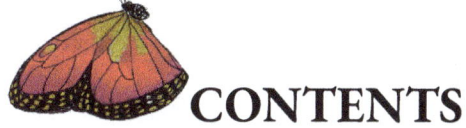
CONTENTS

Prologue……………………………………………………………………7

Chapter One: Understanding Our Unique History………………14

Chapter Two: Acknowledging Our "Choice(s)"
and the Forces Behind Them……………………………………….33

Chapter Three: Recognizing Our Wounds……………………….44

Chapter Four: Understanding Our Pain………………………….58

Chapter Five: Dealing With The Anger…………………………..77

Chapter Six: Grieving Our Losses…………………………………89

Chapter Seven: Forgiving the Unforgivable……………………..99

Chapter Eight: Restoring Hope……………………………………110

Chapter Nine: Walking in Freedom………………………………118

Epilogue……………………………………………………………….129

Addendum: Abortion Proofing Our Children……………………130

References……………………………………………………………135

Sylvia Blakely 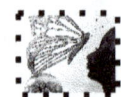 Arise, And Fly Free!

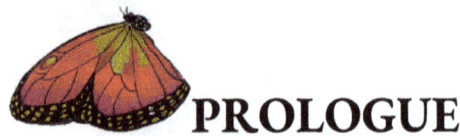 PROLOGUE

January 22, 2022,

I happened to be lying in a borrowed bed in a beautifully appointed Airbnb next to my husband and best friend (same person!) when I was struck like a bolt of lightning. What I heard was, *"Write this down. This will be the beginning of a post-abortion healing curriculum for African American women."*

Now, I've been walking with the Lord long enough to know I'd better answer His call. I grabbed my phone and immediately began to type what was being poured into me. *"Why me? Why now Lord? Was it because I was in Washington, D.C. for my first March for Life which had been so impactful? Was it because a vital segment of the post-abortive population needed to be seen, heard and healed in a way designed specifically for them?"* Whatever His reasons, I knew enough not to ignore them. And so I dictated all that I'd heard spoken. It was way more than I could have imagined on my own.

Ninety minutes later I had the seeds for this healing curriculum. I shared my idea the next morning with Cherilyn Holloway, the friend who asked me to come to Washington in the first place. And then I.did.nothing.for.a.year.

"Great idea Lord, but I don't think I'm ready to deliver it."

So, He got me ready (or should I humbly admit, better prepared!). During 2022, I: **click links to learn more**
- facilitated two sexual abuse classes for SAVAnon (Sexual Abuse Victims Anonymous) with [Sexually Related Trauma Services](#) (SRT) staff;

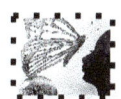

- received training as a facilitator in two healing curricula: *Forgiven and Set Free* written by Linda Cochrane, and *Transforming Your Story* written by Wendy Giancola;
- took a generational trauma course taught by Chandra White-Cummings;
- shepherded women through *SAVEONE*, a five day post-abortion mini curriculum;
- facilitated and participated in an Unravelled Roots book club written by Support After Abortion;
- keynote spoke at Celebration of Restoration, an abortion recovery event in Columbus, OH;
- hosted our first Arise Daughter Gallery Art Show and Wellness Event also in Columbus;
- coordinated a summit on the trauma caused by abortion pills;
- intervened with a group of post-abortive women, led by She Found His Grace in Mississippi, by giving our testimony (Click to hear) in order to shut down the last abortion facility in the state;
- authored my first book for children, featuring The Monarch Butterfly family, which champions Whole Life issues;
- started working with the AND (&) Campaign to produce videos through the Whole Life Project;
- mentored ten women;
- participated in a Deeper Still post-abortion healing retreat in Tampa and a spiritual warfare retreat in Arkansas for ministry leaders;
- shared my testimony and poetry live in D.C while supporting Pro-Black, Pro-Life founder Cherilyn Holloway, and on video for LiveAction (with 125,000 views to date);
- was interviewed by Support After Abortion and Heartbeat International for their podcasts;
- hosted our YouTube channel, Celebrate Life;
- co-facilitated three healing trauma art classes and team lead our ministries, Arise Daughter and Arise Artists.

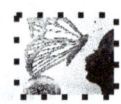

None of this is to brag, trust me. It was all a spiritual boot camp of sorts. I had no more excuses. It was time to shepherd what God had entrusted to me.

I pray this offering hits the mark for a people group that has a unique history with reproductive rights in this country. Our unparalleled experiences will find a space here and be the backdrop for the healing that God wants for all of us.

Is it the be-all and end-all guide? No. But it is humbly presented as the gift it was conceived to be: a loving acknowledgement to the fullness of our experiences as African American women. You will find my story woven through some of the chapters as both a cautionary tale and an example of what God can do with a woman who said "yes" to healing. It is also my way of saying I am "all in" when it comes to supporting you through your healing journey.

If you are using the electronic copy of the curriculum you will find links to songs and other material that will enhance your journey. Click on the links as you see them and allow the material to minister to you. Here are three powerful songs to get you started: (By the way, when you see a reference/link to a song, feel free to listen to it at ANY time during your week. The songs should minister to you as you go about other activities).

- "Believe For It" by CeCe Winans.
- "It's Your Breath In My Lungs" by Todd Galberth.
- "This is The Air I Breathe" by Byron Cage.

Know that this healing journey is a marathon and not a sprint. You didn't get stuck overnight; freedom from the muck will take time, energy and the power of Holy Spirit. If you are working through this alone, might I gently suggest focusing on no more than one chapter per week and enlisting the help of a trusted counselor, pastor or minister to come alongside you. Be sure to pace yourself, take your time and do not skip over or rush through any of the readings or assignments; they will all work together for good. At the end of the study there will be a beautiful time of reflection to remember and honor our children which we call, "The Memorial." More on that later...

If you are in a small group, resist the urge to work ahead. Focus on staying in the present moment and keep in touch with your facilitator at mutually agreed upon times. It will be helpful to break up the study throughout the week so that you are not overwhelmed. If you are doing this alone, know that you will always have the support of Arise Daughter throughout your journey. Feel free to reach out to us at: AriseDaughter@gmail.com for questions regarding the material and to help you get unstuck; that is our calling.

Let's start by fortifying your heavenly connections so that healing can flow. You can connect with God by planning to spend time daily with Him through reading, studying His Word, praying, and worshiping. Helpful resources include: Our Daily Bread, YouVersion Bible, Blue Letter Bible and The Urban Alternative Ministries. There are also several helpful apps you might consider downloading to prompt prayer time such as Pray. Instrumental Soaking Music can also place you in a mood to write and pray.

Plan to notify safe, _trusted_ people in your life like, your mom, grandma, sister, auntie, pastor or women's ministry leader, a prayer partner and your spouse or significant other about the healing journey you will be embarking upon. You WILL need support, a shoulder to cry on and a battle buddy over these next several weeks. Plan to meet with your prayer partner (which is someone you can be accountable to) on a weekly basis and be sure to reach out to them when you feel extra stuck.

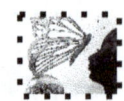

Stray emotions and triggers (sights, sounds and smells that cause a strong emotional response) are bound to show up during your healing. You may also experience dreams that may seem odd as more information about your abortion is revealed. Crafty lies from the enemy of your soul will also break in; be spiritually aware, prepared and prayed up! The Holy Spirit is gentle and kind so, if a stray thought or emotion comes in consider this: is it *convicting* or is it *condemning?* Holy Spirit will reveal or convict you of things so that you can repent and walk closer to God. The enemy invades with thoughts that try to condemn you and draw you AWAY from God. Take each thought captive and examine it carefully through prayer.

Put together a tailor-made *Wellness Plan* for yourself. What is a Wellness Plan? It is a *basket of goodies* that you can go to in the days, hours and minutes when the healing journey gets tough. Your plan could include:

- taking walks
- reading
- spending time in your favorite environment
- gardening
- listening to uplifting music (Arise Daughter on Spotify).

Plan to take care of <u>you</u> these next several weeks by protecting your healing journey. God will meet you where you are and carry you through. Arise Daughter also has a Virtual Wellness Basket on Canva that you can access any time to give you helpful suggestions on how to not only care for yourself but also build your relationship with God.

Another useful strategy is journaling which can be an important outlet for your feelings. You can begin by using a secure notes app on your phone or you can purchase something pretty to write in. Click here for "How to Keep a Spiritual Journal."

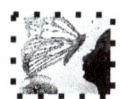

Consider spending time with friends and time alone. Listen to godly preaching and teaching to fortify you. Laugh at whatever you find funny to improve your mood. Put on praise music and sing and dance like only God is watching. You might also head to your favorite coffee or tea spot to watch people. Whatever it is, do it with the intention of increasing your wellbeing and sense of peace.

Be sure to set aside time to simply *feel* all of your raw emotions. Feeling is something that we have to consciously give ourselves permission to do as black women. You don't want to miss anything that God has for your healing journey by shutting your emotions down. Stay as present and in the moment as you can and remember to BREATHE! Refrain from alcohol or other substances that can blunt your emotions while you are on this healing journey. Get adequate sleep and take naps when possible.

Add a creative activity such as [adult coloring](#) at bedtime to calm your mind. Take baths, burn your favorite candle and maybe treat yourself to a massage. Be sure to eat healthy and drink plenty of water. Get outside and let the warmth of the sun nourish you. Did I already mention singing and dancing freely while worshiping God? Keep that strategy on repeat! ([click here for the Arise Daughter Spotify Channel](#) to inspire you).

Set healthy boundaries in certain relationships (you know which ones, "smile"...). ([See these IGs on why boundaries matter part 1](#), [part 2](#)). Practice using the word, *NO* when you simply don't have the bandwidth to handle someone else's drama or some other task ([See this TikTok on effective ways to say *no*](#)). My sister, it is OK to say no to everyone but God while you are healing. AND it is OK to not feel OK as you walk through the valley; Jesus is with you as your Good Shepherd and God is bigger than your heart!

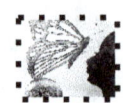

Here is what you can expect from the curriculum: Each chapter will have an historical component, a biblical character reference, the Word of God regarding the chapter topic, an opportunity to check in with yourself and your emotions, hyperlinks to videos, music, books, other readings, social media clips, a time for sharing and reflecting, an art exercise, journaling, prayer and a short but thoughtful homework assignment for the following week. Plan to break up the work throughout the week to give yourself time to go deep. Go back over a section if needed to allow yourself time to process the information. Give yourself and your emotions permission to settle before moving on. Pray when you want understanding or revelation and wait with expectancy for Holy Spirit to reveal the answers you need when you are ready. Let the following verses anchor you as you get started:

"And I am certain that God, who began the good work within you, will continue his work until it is finally finished on the day when Christ Jesus returns."
Philippians 1:6 New Living Translation (NLT)

3 LORD, if you kept a record of our sins, who, O Lord, could ever survive? 4 But you offer forgiveness, that we might learn to fear you. 5 I am counting on the LORD; yes, I am counting on him. I have put my hope in his word.
Psalm 130:3-5

He heals the brokenhearted and bandages their wounds.
Psalm 147:3

Do not be afraid or discouraged, for the LORD will personally go ahead of you. He will be with you; he will neither fail you nor abandon you.
Deuteronomy 31:8

Breathe...and let's get started ladies!

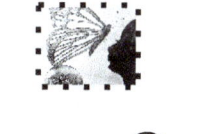

Chapter One

Understanding Our Unique History

"Ain't I A Woman?"
Speech by Sojourner Truth
Click the underlined link to hear the audio and read the speech

Black women have a long and storied history on this planet. Many creationists and evolutionists agree that the first couple who walked the earth were most likely of African origin. That said, oftentimes we start to tell our own story from a purely American point of view without taking into consideration the depth and breadth of our existence or our full value and worth in God's eyes.

From a purely American viewpoint, our "worth" as human beings was inextricably tied to our ability to bear new free labor. Generation after generation experienced a complete and utter disdain for the sanctity of life and family bonds. It simply did not matter to those who enslaved us who fathered our children; how old we were when we were forced to start having children; whether or not we wanted children; nor who might ultimately be responsible for raising our children. In short, for nearly 300 years, we had no free will when it came to childbearing or childrearing; only our fertility mattered. The concept of "family" became very fluid as biological families were torn apart for the commercial advantage of our enslavers.

The abhorrent conditions enslaved people were subjected to, including the rape of both women and men…., the calculated malnourishment and starvation…., the beatings…., the selling of the enslaved…., and the incessant overworking……, meant that we have a lot of trauma to acknowledge as a people and as a nation.

For a more in depth understanding, please read:
- The first person account of slavery: *Incidents in the Life of a Slave Girl* for free on Google Books and Librivox free audio;
- Frederick Douglass' biography: *Narrative of the Life of Frederick Douglass* (Librivox audio and free text);
- Solomon Northup's account of his enslavement in *"12 Years A Slave"*;
- The brief article from encyclopediavirginia.org which recounts the sexual exploitation of enslaved people.

It is a lot to take in so, take your time absorbing it all.

Geneticists such as Richard D. Francis, in his book *Epigenetics: How Environment Shapes Our Genes*, are beginning to recognize that the effects of repeated physical and psychological trauma such as malnutrition and environmental stressors leave lasting damage to the DNA of oppressed people groups. This genetic damage may contribute to all kinds of diseases as genetic alterations are known to last for generations.

Once our hard fought for freedom was granted through the emancipation proclamation of 1865-67, four million black people were turned out of forced servitude with nowhere to go. In a cruel twist, many families eventually settled into sharecropping the land of former enslavers which kept them in poverty. One effective tool used to control the black male population immediately after emancipation was the mass incarceration of "vagrants." This meant that black men who didn't want to sharecrop or had no job prospects could be labeled as "vagrants" and legally moved into the newly enlarged penal system. This strategically planned tactic was meant to separate black men from the family unit yet again thus weakening it. Each state quickly enacted laws after emancipation to create a new way of ensuring cheap labor for state building programs which allowed southern states to continue to build wealth off the bodies of black people.

Some families worked hard to secure land of their own. Having a large family who could farm the land together was a way of keeping food on the table and making sure that the family legacy continued. The trick became how to live peaceably amongst folks who had previously owned you and didn't value or see your inherent worth. Former enslavers who watched those formerly enslaved prosper often went on terrorist sprees which, in some cases leveled whole communities. (For a look into this part of the nation's history, the movie teasers for [Mudbound](), [Black Wall Street Burning]() and [Rosewood]() are great examples to check out.)

This new and uncharted landscape became extremely difficult and often fatal for black folks to navigate. (Listen to a reading of the [Red Record: Tabulated Statistics and Alleged Causes of Lynching in the United States]() by Ida B. Wells-Barnett or read: [On Lynchings]() also by Ms. Wells-Barnett). The Emancipation Proclamation couldn't automatically change a long-standing and ingrained caste system that devalued whole people groups as author Isabel Wilkerson detailed in her two books: [Warmth of Other Suns]() and [Caste](). Both books described the historical basis for the oppression and terrorism of Africans in America and gave context to the antebellum era. Beginning in the early 20th century, millions of black people escaped from the terrorists in the south in an effort to simply live free. This mass migration of millions of people forever changed the landscape of our country.

As large families moved northward, finding adequate housing became an issue. Oftentimes, large families came north in waves with the father going first to secure employment and lodging, then the mother and children coming later. The new northern families' homes often entertained southern relatives wishing to move north to "better themselves," and thus the migration of millions became self-sustaining and family financed. Scores of black families can still mark their migration history by which children were born "down south" and which children were born "up north."

Well into the 1960's, it was rare to see families with fewer than five children. It didn't matter that there may have been only two or three bedrooms and one bathroom in most of the modest homes black folks could afford. Family was family and somehow those large families managed to make it work!

But it became apparent to the new black northerners that the cost of urban living was often prohibitive to raising large families. There was no farm produce or livestock that families could rely on to keep food costs down like in the south. This left many families living paycheck to paycheck: entire households were often tossed to and fro by the whims of fickle employers and landlords.

The black family began to encroach upon the white northerners once black people began to accumulate wealth and buy homes. Tensions surrounding jobs and adequate housing grew as redlining and grandfather clauses barring black home ownership in certain neighborhoods were police-enforced. Segregation created ghettos which persisted well into the 1980's. It was a strange and cold new environment Southern and Northern blacks were entering into where the rules of engagement with whites were unknowable and precarious.

Over time, the lucrative northern manufacturing jobs that African Americans were initially needed for shifted overseas and masses of humanity were left to find low-wage, low-impact jobs. As a result, housing equity, which was and still is the main means to building generational wealth in America, was lost as many people could no longer afford to purchase homes.

Family systems began to fracture as drugs and a second wave of mass incarcerations took their toll on the men who, just a decade before, represented the proud black homeowner and civic participant. Now neighborhoods and mores broke down like never before. The black church, being unable to keep up with the swift and massive changes, became insular and isolated as they were overwhelmed with the societal shifts. White flight and then middle class black flight left our cities decimated and more like impenetrable war zones. Many folks who were left in poverty felt like their only choice was to *get out* of the ghettos and move into the suburbs where they found that they most assuredly were NOT welcomed.

Into this societal chaos and confusion slides Margaret Sanger and her selective population control ideas. The practice of Eugenics or "good genes" was meant to weed out those she and others decided were no longer fit to breed. Ms. Sanger had aligned herself early on with rich and powerful northerners like John D. Rockefeller who were willing to bankroll the development of various forms of birth control. Mr. Rockefeller and other elites were also concerned about being overwhelmed by the sheer number of southern blacks migrating north. These population control plans collided with the hardships of life in the north for second generation black migrants. What started out as a deliberate plan to limit the size of black families morphed into a casual conversation about helping negro women out of their reproductive "mess."

Black women began to become interested in limiting family size out of financial necessity and lack of employment opportunities fueled by carefully marketed population control rhetoric. This is when the evil of the abortion movement began in earnest. Ideas put forth by eugenicists for controlling the birth rate of blacks using forced sterilization had limited success and drew unwanted attention (read Dorothy Roberts' *Killing the Black Body*.)

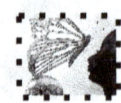

When it became difficult to sell eugenics (especially after World War II and all that happened to the Jews in Nazi Germany) population control methods were repackaged as *"planning parenthood" by Ms. Sanger*. Leaders such as W.E.B DuBois joined in this movement with the aim of giving black women control over their bodies through the availability and use of birth control. On the surface, this made sense. Historically, black women had little choice about anything. The lure of controlling *your own reproductive destiny* was used by Sanger and her fledgling organization, the American Birth Control League (which later became Planned Parenthood), to evoke a fake sense of personal freedom. Meanwhile, Planned Parenthood hid for decades their racist underlying agenda of reducing the number of black births. My sister, it was a set-up from the beginning. Are you seeing it?

"The most successful educational approach to the Negro is through a religious appeal. We do not want word to go out that we want to exterminate the Negro population, and the Minister is the man who can straighten out that idea if it ever occurs to any of their more rebellious members."
– *Margaret Sanger, Eugenicist and founder of Planned Parenthood*

Thinly veiled attempts to keep the black population from growing were shunned by black leadership of the day. In fact, few in the black community saw government-sanctioned population management as a good idea; after all, there had been enough of that kind of control in the earliest history of this country amongst all minority groups. Leaders in the black community such as Marcus Garvey, Ms. Fannie Lou Hammer, Dr. Martin Luther King, The Nation of Islam, the Black Panthers and prominent Black pastors heard what was really being said underneath the Planned Parenthood rhetoric which was: *If you can control the population of the poor and other "undesirables", you keep them powerless.*

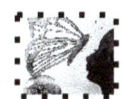

In steps Congress and the formation of the United States Office of Population Affairs (OPA), which was established in 1970, to regulate population growth especially among low-income families. This move brought legislative clout and urban development dollars to the mix. Peruse their website today and you will be able to find the telling statement that, "OPA and the Title X program is designed to provide access to contraceptive services, supplies, and information. By law, priority is given to persons from low-income families." This was all under the guise of *healthcare access for the poor*; what it actually did was fund Planned Parenthood's services. (Title X Program Funding History | HHS Office of Population Affairs)

The newly revamped Democratic Party (which flipped from conservative white southerners to liberal white northerners) in the 60's tied themselves to organizations such as Planned Parenthood because they seemed to be on the same bandwagon as other groups fighting for *human rights*. Reproductive control slowly morphed into reproductive *rights* which stuck as part of a new agenda. And where did all of this new Title X government money pour into? The black community which was desperate for revitalization and access to services. The wolf was dressed in lambskin and invited to eat at the economic redevelopment table. Segregated cities, with limited access to physicians, became easy targets for *"health clinics"* and the *"right"* to reproductive services, including abortion, was spawned.

The pervasive and persuasive subliminal messages embedded in Planned Parenthood literature were:

Plan when YOU want to parent which is your right. Here are the government-funded tools to allow you to regain control over YOUR destiny. Have children when YOU are ready and not a minute before. Consider abortion to be the same as contraception: a simple and safe procedure - just like any other medical procedure. In fact, you won't need to be hospitalized or risk a back alley hack. We can perform abortion on-demand in the comfort of your own

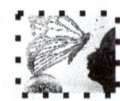

neighborhood "health center" and have you back at work within a few days. Come back as many times as you can afford - it is your right to do so and the costs will always be subsidized as long as Title X is in place.

What Planned Parenthood REALLY meant was, *we don't want YOUR kind reproducing*. Yes, you read that last sentence right. From its beginning Planned Parenthood's agenda has been to limit the reproduction of the *negro and other undesireables*. Their true goal has always been population control in certain neighborhoods. Why was their agenda eventually co-opted by religious leaders and parishioners alike? Because the eugenics message was masterfully rebranded as "health care" in underserved communities by Ms. Sanger. Why did we, as Christians, allow God to have little or nothing to say about our purity, holiness and reproduction? Because we wanted control over this aspect of our lives.

Does any of this ring true for you? It did for MANY African American Christian women and men. Not only was the lure of economic mobility for a people who had experienced multi-generational poverty too much to ignore, but the sin of spilling innocent blood was largely brushed aside by some ministers and medical professionals who convinced us that "it" was only a "blob of tissue" without significance. It's no wonder we took the carefully wrapped bait.

Financial difficulties have traditionally topped the list of reasons why many women, even Christian women, chose abortion even when they didn't want to. We never had an infrastructure in place to support our pregnancies other than during slavery. The church was conflicted when it came to caring for the single pregnant woman. There were many congregations back in the day, who would shame a young woman in front of the whole church, if she was found to be pregnant out of wedlock. Many girls were sent "down south" for various made-up reasons before their pregnant belly started to show so that they could have their babies in secret. Countless children have been raised as a "cousin" to their own biological mother. Please know that there is no condemnation in understanding the *'why'* of our *choice(s)*. Let us recognize, however, that relatively few government funds actually went towards helping families with an unexpected pregnancy even when that was the desire of the parent's heart. Isn't that curious? Putting it in the most basic terms, the government was willing to help me terminate my child and not so willing to help me parent my child because it is cheaper to abort a child than to raise it. In short but, to the point, the state sees an unplanned pregnancy as a drain to its resources even as the parents of that child pay taxes to support the state.

Once the propaganda made the child out to be the *crisis* and not the limited bank account or resources, it set up an *either/or* scenario. The underlying message was, *Keep your child and stay poor OR abort your child and gain financial freedom*. If we don't catch this subtlety, then we miss how the abortion-mill rhetoric managed to pit women against their unborn children in a society where capitalism has become the newest idol.

After Roe v. Wade was ensconced into law - equating abortion with the right to privacy - we could not only abort our children legally, but we could also keep our secret(s). We were clearly in the grip of the oldest enemy of humankind which is Satan, and his familiar tactics. Yes, the same one that comes to lie (John 8:44), and steal, kill and destroy (John 10:10) got a foothold into our families. The practice of child sacrifice, as in the nations that practiced it millenia ago (2 Chronicles 28:3), became the accepted - no - expected behavior of a new, *free* generation in America. What was legal versus what was moral were disconnected from each other and we spiraled out of control.

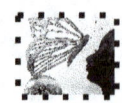

We were now *free* and had the legal *right* to kill our own children whenever and however we wanted. I acknowledge and recognize that for some very young women, the *choice* to keep or abort their child was outside of their control. We also have to acknowledge that after 1973, the government did in fact give tacit permission to *some adult* in that young person's life to sign for an abortion that they felt was in the best interest of the minor. Either way, we do want to recognize that everyone's abortion story is different; the one common factor is that our children are gone...

The prophet Jeremiah spoke of the sins of the nation of Israel towards the innocent children of his time. Jeremiah 19:4-5 states: 4 *"For Israel has forsaken me and turned this valley into a place of wickedness. The people burn incense to foreign gods--idols never before acknowledged by this generation, by their ancestors, or by the kings of Judah. And they have filled this place with the blood of innocent children. 5 They have built pagan shrines to Baal, and there they burn their sons as sacrifices to Baal. I have never commanded such a horrible deed; it never even crossed my mind to command such a thing!*

God, in His benevolence, was trying to get Israel to see the sin they were committing against children. Psalms 94: 6-7 They kill widows and foreigners and murder orphans. 7 "The LORD isn't looking," they say, "and besides, the God of Israel doesn't care."

God DOES CARE and He is STILL trying to get our attention as it relates to the health and safety of His smallest image bearers.

Through all of the societal upheavals of this nation, God continued to keep His eye on us! Just like the captives in Egypt and Babylon, God purposed us to "be fruitful and multiply" (Exodus 1:7), bless not curse our new home (Jeremiah 29:4-15) and continue to look for His rescuing arm (Jeremiah 23:3). The caveat is that we must first recognize that what we have allowed society to dictate to us about the lives of our preborn children was and is wrong.

The preborn have been planned for by God (Jeremiah 29:11), and new parents have responsibilities (Titus 2:4; Isaiah 49:15). Once that realization sinks in, there is no limit to how God can bless His people when we return to Him and put our faith and trust in Him regarding procreation (2 Chronicles 6:38; Jeremiah 23:3-8; 24:6-7).

These next 8-9 weeks will be focused on recognizing, repenting and reconciling our *choices*. It will be heavy work, and I highly recommend that you enlist support from someone you trust who can lift you up through the process. Note that the word *process* is used. This healing journey most likely will be multi-layered like an onion. Tears will be shed as layers of painful lies are removed, not only for you, but for the millions that have gone before you. But remember beloved, you're here because you know there is unfinished business to attend to in order to be reconciled with God regarding your abortion(s).

This guide to healing was designed to be used in a small group setting, however, if you do decide to work at your own pace, know that Holy Spirit can and will see you through. Your sisters at Arise Daughter are also available to serve as mentors when and if you need us!

Consider this: 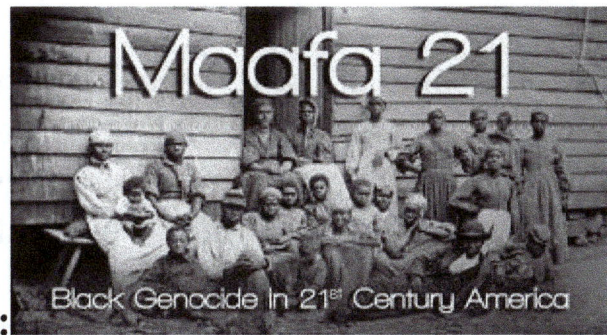 Maafa 21: Black Genocide in 21st Century America (full documentary).

- What were two *takeaways* from the video that left an impression?

This is a good place to take a break and process. Take your time. Continue when you are ready with
Chapter 1 part B.

 ### What Does God Have to Say?

Let's take a look at God's character. God's desire has always been to have a loving and intimate relationship with His creation and that includes each one of us. He created man in His image to commune with Him in a unique and loving way. The God we serve is the only wise God (Romans 16:27). Our God has dominion and power over ALL of the earth and its creation (Jude 1:25) and yet He chose us to share who He is more fully. As we think about some of the ways God can manifest Himself to us and show His love for us, it can be both comforting and overwhelming. If we allow ourselves to rest in the fact that God truly loves and wants what is best for us then that knowledge allows us to let God be God in every aspect of our lives (Psalm 146:5-10).

But, let's be honest: For some of us, it has been difficult to relinquish control over our lives - even to an all knowing and generous God. There may be many reasons for this. For example, some of our reasons may come from past experiences with our own father or a surrogate father. Many of us have "father wounds" which may make it difficult to see God as the loving Father that He is. Some of us may be holding on to negative belief systems and patterns learned in childhood or that are generational in nature.

God's character is independent of us in that He is "I AM." We don't define God, but we do try to better understand who He is through our relationship with Him. Our relationship with Him is built through His Word, through following His Son Jesus and through fellowship with Holy Spirit. God is an all seeing God and, yes beloved, He sees you right where you are. He knows your brokenness and He is the God who is able to bind up all of your wounds. Psalms 147: 3 AMP says, He heals the brokenhearted and binds up their wounds [healing their pain and comforting their sorrow.]

He wants you to take the time to get to know HIM better. He wants to build a new intimate bond with you; one where you can learn to love Him, trust Him in every aspect of your life and understand His will for your life. This intimacy requires knowledge of who our heavenly Father is and His character; that is what we will look at next.

Below is a list of some of the names for God. As you read each name carefully, make a note of which name speaks most to you in this season. In God's names, we clearly see His character. An additional resource to learn more about God's character would be the BibleProject.com video series on the "Character of God" which is HIGHLY recommended (click HERE to view on YouTube).

Notes on the video:

The Names of God (Not an exhaustive list. From open sources)

Names of God	Meanings
Yahweh-YHWH-Jehovah (in English)	I am; He that is; He who makes that which has been made.
El-Shaddai	Lord God almighty
El-Elyon	The most High God
Adonai	Lord, Master
Elohim	God
El Roi	The God who sees me
Abba	Father
Magen	The Lord is my shield
Jehovah Nissi	The Lord my banner
Jehovah Raah	The Lord my shepherd
Jehovah Rapha	The Lord that heals
Jehovah Shammah	The Lord is there
Jehovah Tsidkenu	The Lord our righteousness
Jehovah Mekoddishkem	The Lord who sanctifies you
Jehovah Jireh	The Lord will provide
Jehovah Shalom	The Lord is peace
Jehovah Sabaoth	The Lord of hosts
Jehovah Makkeh	The Lord who strikes
Jehovah Tsuri	The Lord is my rock

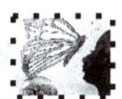

God is patient and kind and He has always sought the best for us despite our sins (or the sins committed against us). His original intention was for us to be fruitful and to populate the earth with more image bearers with whom He could form loving relationships with. He wants us to care for His creation as He has cared for us; but we all know how original sin messed THAT up! We also know that we serve a God that can make beauty from ashes (Isaiah 61:3). God's intention has been to restore us to our original state of being in intimate communion with Him and, that is why His son was sent (John 3:16-17). More on that later...

For now, let us focus on the first command, which was a blessing for all of creation: (*highlight any words in the following verses that stand out to you*).

Then God blessed them, saying, "Be fruitful and multiply. Let the fish fill the seas, and let the birds multiply on the earth."
Genesis 1:22

- After God declared all He'd made was good, what does God say to His new creation?

- What purpose(s) did God have for speaking to His creation?

26 Then God said, "Let us make human beings in our image, to be like us. They will reign over the fish in the sea, the birds in the sky, the livestock, all the wild animals on the earth, and the small animals that scurry along the ground." 27 So God created human beings in his own image. In the image of God he created them; male and female he created them. 28 Then God blessed them and said, "Be fruitful and multiply. Fill the earth and govern it. Reign over the fish in the sea, the birds in the sky, and all the animals that scurry along the ground."
Genesis 1:26-28

- The verses remind us that God created us in His image to be good and to do good. What comfort does that bring to you?

- As you consider these verses, was "multiplying" meant to be a blessing? Why?

<u>Bible connection</u>: Consider God's first human female-Eve-and the promises God made to her. In Genesis 3:16 God told Eve that she will desire and long for her husband (husband is defined as the person she was sexually intimate with). This reminds us that God ordained women to want to : a. Become "one" with only one husband B. desire our own husbands sexually and C. Be fruitful and bear children that would have dominion over the earth. There is tremendous promise for Eve and her offspring despite the fall. God promises that one of her offspring (Jesus) would crush the serpent that tricked her. <u>Reflection</u>: God always has a plan of redemption ready even when we mess up and sometimes, that plan involves our offspring.

I will make you extremely fruitful. Your descendants will become many nations, and kings will be among them!
Genesis 17:6

- What important promises were made to Abram and Sarai regarding their offspring?

Meanwhile, the people of Israel settled in the region of Goshen in Egypt. There they acquired property, and they were fruitful, and their population grew rapidly.
Genesis 47:27

- Why is it significant to look at <u>where</u> Israel prospered?

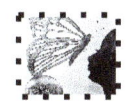

3 Your wife [shall be] like a fruitful vine in the very heart of your house, your children like olive plants all around your table. 4 Behold, thus shall the man be blessed who fears the LORD. 6 Yes, may you see your children's children. Peace [be] upon Israel!"
Psalm 128:3-4, 6 NASB

- What is God calling us to look and live like in the verses above?

- How is the blessing generational?

4 Remain in me, and I will remain in you. For a branch cannot produce fruit if it is severed from the vine, and you cannot be fruitful unless you remain in me. 5 "Yes, I am the vine; you are the branches. Those who remain in me, and I in them, will produce much fruit. For apart from me you can do nothing.
John 15:4-5

- As you interpret this verse, where does the source of our strength come from?

- Which of the names of God (from the table above) apply best to the verses in John 15?

- In conclusion, are we designed to make a life outside of God and His original intention for us? Why not?

Check In: "Visualizing The Lord's Prayer" (Click on the link to see how to effectively pray the "Lord's prayer").

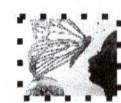

Pray, then, in this way: 'Our Father, who is in heaven, Hallowed be Your name. Your kingdom come, Your will be done on earth as it is in heaven. Give us this day our daily bread. And forgive us our debts, as we have forgiven our debtors [letting go of both the wrong and the resentment]. And do not lead us into temptation, but deliver us from evil. [For Yours is the kingdom and the power and the glory forever. Amen.}
Matthew 6:9-13 AMP

==What are your thoughts, feelings and emotions about starting this journey?==

Share in the group or feel free to journal what you are feeling. Take your time and allow your thoughts to flow. Try your best not to censor or edit what you write.

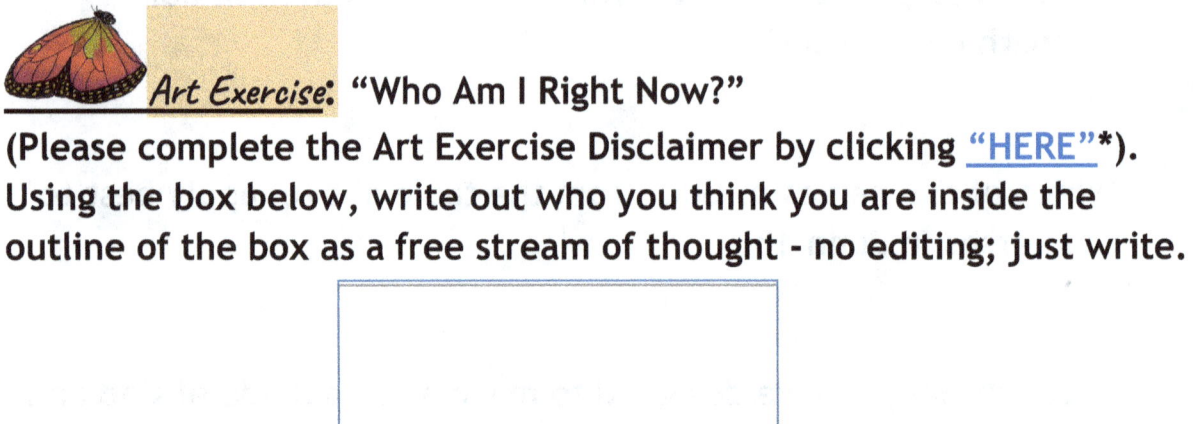

(Please complete the Art Exercise Disclaimer by clicking "HERE"*). Using the box below, write out who you think you are inside the outline of the box as a free stream of thought - no editing; just write.

Write Out Your Prayer

Let God know what you now understand about the lies you were told, or simply talk to God about what it feels like to start this healing journey. What name of God or characteristic could you add in your prayer? Include three things in your prayer that you are grateful for.

Songs (Remember to allow the music to minister to you).

- "I Don't Feel Noways Tired" by Peter Collins and Infinity Song.
- "I Don't Feel Noways Tired" by Rev. James Cleveland.
- "Deep Enough" by Anthony Brown.
- "Breathe" by Maverick City Music

Homework

Take the "Feelings" Journey, courtesy of New Life Ministries. Print your results or screen shot them if possible. Activate your Wellness Plan.

Notes:

Chapter Two

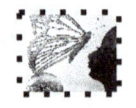

Acknowledging Our "Choice(s)" and the Forces Behind Them

> *"The prime condition of slavery was to keep closed every avenue to knowledge. The Negro had no estate, no family life. His sole inheritance was his body."*
> Booker T. Washington

Our choices have history. We were a people group prized for our ability to work hard and to breed. It sounds harsh, but the wealth of the early Americas was literally built through the wombs of African women. The right to our wombs was bought and paid for by European landowners who then codified into law in the 1600's that any progeny would hold the bond status of its mother, thus perpetuating servitude (Read: "Learning for Justice").

Girls were chosen for rape and breeding as soon as their menstrual cycles (which were closely monitored by their owners) began. Once the importation of slaves was legally halted in the 1860's, enslavers had to solely rely on the breeding of enslaved women. It didn't matter whether or not there was any feeling between the pair chosen for breeding or even if there was a familial tie. And if the enslaver could reliably father his own bondservants without giving the resulting children any rights, then all the better. Enslavers went so far as to enact laws that made the rape of black women a statutory impossibility (Rape As A Badge Of Slavery: The Legal History Of, And Remedies For, Prosecutorial Race-Of-Victim Charging Disparities by Jeffrey J. Pokorak). The echoes of laws like this still reverberate. Black women are often seen as, "loose" and

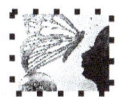

"asking" for the sexual violence perpetrated against them. Again, we see how the enemy can twist an evil thought, make it law and attempt to take away the evil intention.

Did enslaved women have ANY choice in childbearing? Of course not. How did black men feel about being denied the opportunity to marry for love, not having exclusive marriage bed rights, being forced to breed like livestock and being sold away from their families of origin? Has anyone bothered to ask them? The immensity of the moral crimes is huge, make no mistake.

Walk forward to the 1930's when reproductive *freedom* felt real and tangible for black women truly for the first time. According to Dorothy Roberts in *Killing the Black Body*, contraceptive clinics were being established in major urban areas like Harlem, NY with the support of luminaries such as W.E.B DuBois who were vocal about supporting birth control and a woman's right to motherhood at her own discretion as previously mentioned. Freedom to choose when, how, why, and with whom to have sex with was embraced by many, and understandably so. We had just come out of a very long and dark era where we were forced to have sex and to raise the children of our rapist without question or hesitation. We secretly wanted what we thought white women always had, which was reproductive freedom. Black women wanted freedom to not only pick and choose their partners, but also the freedom to determine *when* to have sex and, crucially, *how many* children to have. Of course freedom rarely comes without responsibility. But being *responsible* was never a question. Black women have always been responsible. We were responsible not only for our own but also the children of our enslavers. We were made to be *overly* responsible for everybody else. We were forced to nurse our enslavers' children and let our own go hungry.

Let that sink in. It is not a small thing to acknowledge.

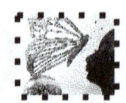

We knew about the private doctors white women could access to *take care of* unplanned pregnancies. We knew because we took care of their households while they were on *medical holiday*. We didn't have that. So, as the Planned Parenthood movement swept into our neighborhoods offering us *access* to birth control and the *choice* to terminate our pregnancy, we became excited by the notion that we could actually have some kinda say. Some of us can remember when the book, *"Our Bodies, Our Choice"* began to circulate in the 1970's; it was both revolutionary and a revelation at the same time. We began to demand rights and abilities in this country that we had never known. Ever. Some of us thought that if we gained parity with white women and removed the power over our bodies from the white man then, Planned Parenthood could help us do just that. After all, it seemed to have the answers we were looking for. Clinics swept into our neighborhoods and became the primary access point for women's "health care." What we didn't know was that doctors were paid cash under the table to perform as many abortions in a day as possible. Never mind that the care Planned Parenthood provided was targeted towards controlling the population of African-Americans. We bought the lie that some attention was better than nothing and we fell under their control.

For some women today, any word against Planned Parenthood is a blow to their personal *freedom of "choice."* Few women and men stop to think, "What 'choices' are they actually providing me with? What are they doing to actually help me *parent* my child?" If you were *"right now old" when* this struck you, take the time to question whether or not you were offered <u>any</u> financial or emotional assistance by the abortion clinic to *actually help you become a parent*. Or, was an abortion presented as the *best* option given your (typically temporary) vulnerable circumstances? Why weren't you offered vouchers for transportation and housing? Why couldn't you get a crib or car seat or diapers or clothes from an agency that had "Parenthood" in their name? The depth of the deception is hard to make sense of. Add to this the warping of the term, "Reproductive Justice" which has been co-opted by many to equate "justice" with the ability to decide which innocent black child dies. It is hard to make any of this make any moral sense but this is the current state of our fallen world.

I believe we truly did not know how devastating our abortion *choice(s)* would be for ourselves and for future generations. I believe the majority of us did not fully understand what an abortion actually involved for our baby or for ourselves. We did not know the lasting effects of hormonal birth control and how that would negatively affect our health in general or our reproductive health specifically. In fact, a [Time magazine article](#) recently pointed to the fact that many women of color were coerced into taking pills and implants which had lasting negative effects on their fertility and their mental health.

My dear Sisters, with over 20 million dead African American babies since 1973, untold cases of sexually transmitted diseases, broken relationships and homes, sex outside of marriage with multiple men fathering multiple children... is it surprising that we are no closer to just treatment for ourselves or our children? Beloved sister, this is not who God designed us to be. We were meant to be more.

I am not pointing out this harsh reality to be condemning AT ALL; quite the contrary! I was as caught up in the rhetoric and lies as much as anybody else. It took me over 20 years to learn that applied knowledge is wisdom. We have to acknowledge the facts of where we've come from and where God wants to move us to. And no matter how difficult it is, if we want to do things God's way and make a different *choice* next time, we have to look closely at how we got here.

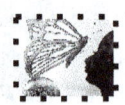

BIBLE CONNECTION: Consider the daughters of Lot (Genesis 19:30-38). They took the unprecedented step of sleeping with their father after the destruction of Sodom and Gomorrah. Their intention was to continue the family bloodline at any cost. In taking matters into their own hands they left God out of their decision making. What came from that was the humiliation of their father and the birth of two pagan nations: the Moabites and the Ammonites who later came to oppose Israel. REFLECTION: Taking matters into your own hands rarely ends well and can have generational implications. Don't just do something: Wait and Ask God for your "next" steps.

 *What Does God Have to Say?*

We were not the first people group to be targeted by enslavers. The Israelites in captivity in Egypt are the group that often comes to mind in comparison. There are so many dissimilar aspects to our two stories, but there is one important similarity as well: God allowed us both to be fruitful and to multiply in greater numbers than our captors. Children have been and always will be a blessing to God despite the circumstances of their birth. Even when we could not control our children's fate, God stepped in time and time again to protect them.

He is the same God now as He was back then.

Have there been instances in your life where you could clearly see the protective hand of God on you and how He shielded you? (The name, Magen-The Lord is my shield would be an important characteristic of God to consider). Take a minute and recount as many instances as you can.

God rules a Kingdom that does not know what "lack" means. Our Heavenly Father has never seen any of us as, "less than" because of the circumstances of our birth, our bank account or anything else. His good intentions for us have never been based upon how others see us. We have to rely on the character of God and who HE is because only God's opinion about us matters. God is ruler over all. He is trustworthy and kind. Our God is reliable, faithful and dependable. Our relationship with Him will last throughout eternity so our focus should always be on His will for our lives. Where man will fail us, God never will! (For spiritual inspiration, read Psalm 139).

In his letter to the church in Galatia, the apostle Paul made one of the boldest and most unifying statements of its time:

There is no longer Jew or Gentile, slave or free, male and female. For you are all one in Christ Jesus.
Galatians 3:28

- What is your understanding of your worth in God's eyes in comparison to others? Did a hardship or trial make you question your worth?

- According to the above verse, where is our worth found?

For we are God's masterpiece. He has created us anew in Christ Jesus, so we can do the good things he planned for us long ago.
Ephesians 2:10

- Does it surprise you that God prepared good works for each of us ahead of time? Why or why not?

- Why do you think God was not surprised by your pregnancy or pregnancies?

- Does God's foreknowledge about His creation impact how you now think of your pregnancy or pregnancies?

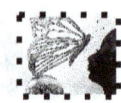

12 But to all who believed him and accepted him, he gave the right to become children of God. 13 They are reborn--not with a physical birth resulting from human passion or plan, but a birth that comes from God.
John 1:12-13

- Looking at this verse, what is your understanding of God's grace as Father and Creator?

- Describe how God partners with us given that we have *free will*.

- Is God bound by what happened in previous generations? Why or why not?

But the person who is joined to the Lord is one spirit with him..
1 Corinthians 6:17

- Going back to your childhood for a moment, did you have a sense of a divine connection with God? At what age? Describe what it felt like.

- Have you ever felt distant from God (the Father), Jesus and/or Holy Spirit?

- Describe a time when you questioned if He could see and hear you? How did that feel?

- Did your abortion(s) take you farther away or move you closer to God? How? Describe in detail.

Don't you realize that your body is the temple of the Holy Spirit, who lives in you and was given to you by God? You do not belong to yourself,
1 Corinthians 6:19

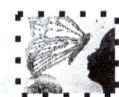

- What is your understanding of what this verse means both for you and for your child(ren) lost to abortion?

- Do you believe in the eternal nature of our spirit/soul? If so, why? If no, why not?

For you are all children of the light and of the day; we don't belong to darkness and night.
1 Thessalonians 5:5

- How did your choice(s) to abort usher in a dark period in your life?

- Did you recognize you were in the darkness? Why or why not?

- What choices did you make afterwards that kept you in darkness?

- Who or what showed up as light for you while you were in that dark place?

3 We are human, but we don't wage war as humans do. 4 We use God's mighty weapons, not worldly weapons, to knock down the strongholds of human reasoning and to destroy false arguments. 5 We destroy every proud obstacle that keeps people from knowing God. We capture their rebellious thoughts and teach them to obey Christ.
2 Corinthians 10:3-5 NLT

- What is the definition of a spiritual stronghold? (The resource, "GotQuestions.org" is helpful in providing definitions).

- What lies from the enemy did you help to reinforce in your mind?

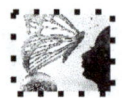

Check In:

Now would be a good time to stop and breathe through our current emotions. (Click to learn a breathing technique called "Box Breathing").

Expert opinion:

- "Generational Trauma" by Dr. Joy DeGruy -One hour
- "Intro. To Post Traumatic Slave Syndrome" by Dr. Joy DeGruy - Five minutes
- "Strangling Strongholds" by Dharius Daniels- 53 minutes

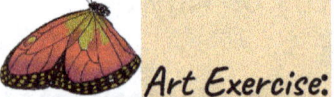 **Art Exercise:** "Generational Influences" Timeline

Create a timeline of events involving as many generations as you can backwards and forwards to examine intergenerational trauma and societal influences on your abortion decision. For example, if family members before you had abortions include them in your timeline. Start with your birth year at the center of the line and work forwards and backwards. Be sure to include significant events that followed your abortion.

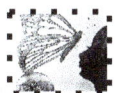

Blank Timeline Template

Title Name: Date:

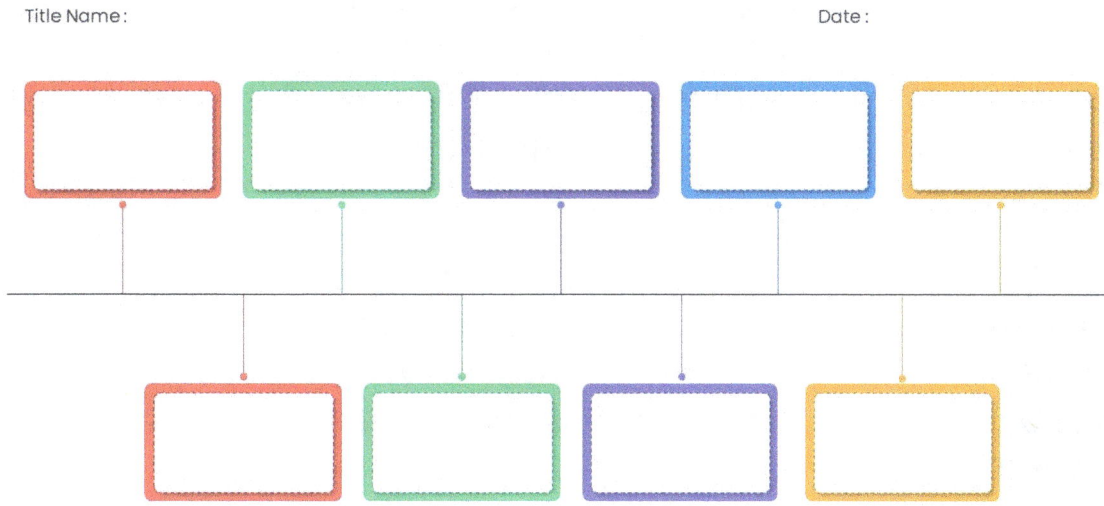

Now let's share our timeline stories.

- How did telling your timeline story make you feel?

- How can you relate to your sister's experience?

- What other factors influenced your choice(s)?

- Can you recognize any repeating negative patterns or strongholds within your family such as divorce, adultery, sex before marriage?

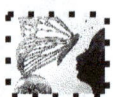

Full Circle Moment of Reflection

Let's take a moment of quiet time to process what we've heard, read and shared thus far. Feel free to share the results of your homework, the *Feelings Journey*, with the group. Allow yourself to journal any thoughts or emotions to help you reflect and process.

Write Your Prayer

If you have never taken your abortion(s) and the darkness you carry to the light of Jesus, do so now as a written prayer. Include a name for God or a characteristic of God in your prayer. Include three things you are grateful for.

Song

- *"Draw Nigh"* by Fred Hammond

Homework: "Who Was I?"

Locate a photograph of you around the age you first felt connected to God. If you don't have a photo, simply sit and visualize yourself at the appropriate age. Write a letter to that younger self for next week. Check in with your Wellness Team.

Chapter 3

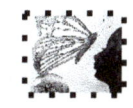

Recognizing Our Wounds

"He who concealers his disease cannot expect to be cured."
African Proverb

The reason you've made it to week three (congratulations by the way!) is because you want to begin to finally acknowledge the wound(s) left by the loss of your child(ren). God meant for us to feel the loss of a child. Society tells us that with an abortion, we haven't really lost anything of value; but our souls know what has taken place. Once our *relief* from the abortion transitions into *regret*, the ugly task of reconciling two different belief systems (God's absolute truth and man's half truths) begins. This is when we need to allow ourselves to recognize our woundedness.

But let's step back a bit... How many significant and traumatic events have we had to push aside in order to simply continue on with the business of living? In her book, *Post Traumatic Slave Syndrome*, Dr. Joy De Gruy outlines the various long-term effects of being, arguably, the most significantly oppressed race in America. Our level of oppression cannot really be measured (nor can anyones), yet her work helps address and make sense of the patterns of behavior we likely misread because of our centuries long oppression. Our day to day interactions with others as well as the self-talk we have become used to are all tainted by years of enslavement. We learned to accept traumatic experiences as a way to persevere yet, in a cruel twist, we have often inflicted trauma on ourselves and others within our race in order to offload the burden of racism.

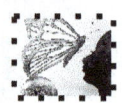

Slavery deeply disrupted the family structure of our African forefathers. Even after emancipation, a calculated program of mass incarceration of our men led to further destruction of traditional family values (read *The New Jim Crow* by Michelle Alexander). As a result, many of us have lived through generations of absentee parents and all that comes with missing out on their love and physical presence. Many of us have also experienced sexual molestation, physical and verbal abuse as well as the systemic racism that caused many of our social ills. The blatant and pernicious racism we've faced both in school and on the job has kept us in "trauma response" mode. When you are simply trying to survive day to day, you learn to quickly triage injury and pain, patch it up, and keep it moving as if you were in a war zone. Past traumas are a huge part of our story however, we never had the luxury of stopping to acknowledge our woundedness until now. There may be voices around you that are still trying to silence you or negate your history; ignore them and keep healing.

For some of us, dealing with the trauma of an absentee father created a lack of understanding of the proper role of men in our lives (including the father of our child(ren) who might also have been dealing with profound loss). When two traumatized people enter into a sexual relationship, the result is sure to be rocky. Recently two young women admitted that they had formed a "trauma bond" with their baby's father basically acknowledging that their past trauma was the common thread in their hookups. After the abortion, neither party had the emotional bandwidth to deal with the aftermath and so the relationships dissolved. Both mother and father are left then to grieve two losses- the baby AND the relationship- which adds to the emotional baggage they were already carrying.

It is often said that the very first step of a healing journey is acknowledging that we have a wound to heal. So few of us get started on a healing journey because, quite frankly, we have invested our time and energy into covering up our wounds. As one sister shared

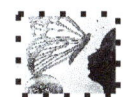

with me, "Who has the time or the emotional energy to talk about my abortion wounds when I'm dealing with so many other traumas?" On top of that, how do you even know if what you are feeling is related to the abortion(s) or to some other past situation? You can easily see how messy healing can be!

We use phrases like, "I'm fine." "I'm so over that" "What's done is done." "It was my fault anyway" to deny or mask our pain. Sometimes, it seems that we either want to be magicians - wishing it all away like nothing significant really happened - or we become judge, jury and executioner of our past selves. In both scenarios, the wounds are left to fester.

What, specifically, do festering abortion wounds look like? If, for example, you thought of your abortion(s) as a physical wound, what would it look like? Spend some time thinking about that and later you will be asked to try to describe with words or a drawing what you imagine.

Post Abortion wounds can manifest themselves in the mind as something known as *Post Abortion Stress Syndrome or PASS*. Symptoms of abortion trauma may include the following: (Circle, underline or highlight those you have experienced. Take your time).

Bouts of crying, *depression*, guilt, *inability to forgive yourself*, intense grief/sadness, anger/rage, emotional numbness, SEXUAL PROBLEMS OR PROMISCUITY, eating disorders, **lowered self-esteem**, drug and alcohol abuse, nightmares and sleep disturbances, suicidal urges, *difficulty with relationships*, anxiety and panic attacks, flashbacks, multiple abortions, pattern of repeat crisis pregnancies, discomfort around babies or pregnant women, *fear/ambivalence of pregnancy* plus others that can affect future parenting. (list compiled by H3Helpline.org)

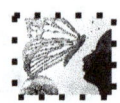

Additionally, emotional triggers such as: suction sounds from machines, heavy bleeding or clots passed during normal periods, annual gynecological check ups, and future pregnancies can also create trauma wounds that can become quite complex to treat.

Be aware that the enemy will try to convince you of one of two things: 1. Acknowledging your post-abortion pain is not really relevant to your *new* life OR 2. You must have had a pre-existing mental health condition if you are struggling with your abortion. There was a research article published by the National Institutes of Health titled: *The abortion and mental health controversy* which acknowledged that women with prior mental health conditions will indeed struggle more after their abortion. For instance, millions of women who suffer with anxiety and depression will have an increase in PASS symptoms after abortion(s).

You might have been told that you are just acting "extra" and that it "doesn't take all that" to "get over" an abortion(s). Your partner or family might complain or feel inconvenienced by your grief. People who respond that way may mean well but, essentially they are canceling your legitimate feelings of loss. You might think you don't have the right to feel "a certain way" or you may be confused by your lack of emotions. The terms that are used to describe this type of pain are, "forbidden grief" and "disenfranchised grief."

There is almost no room made by abortionists for acknowledgement of the mental pain that is most certainly real for many women. It is important to note that one research study titled, "Relief Most Common Emotion 5 years Post-Abortion" has shown that many women initially do feel a sense of relief after a surgical abortion. This relief, however, was only studied five years out from the abortion. Many abortion recovery facilitators know from personal experience that once the numbness wears off (which can take more

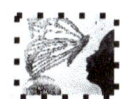

than five years), regret comes to the forefront. In addition, the study does not highlight, for example, the unique trauma experienced by women who take the abortion pills. The emotional trauma caused by chemical abortions is unique since the patient is also her own abortionist and has no real idea of what to expect from the experience nor is she trained to handle the aftermath.

Be wary of anyone who works overtime to minimize or negate your feelings or who doesn't acknowledge your numbness! That person is not in tune with you. You have the right to feel how you feel and no one should be allowed to cancel you or gaslight your feelings. No one.

The majority of women did not expect the emotional fallout that came from exercising our abortion *rights*. We were told that we were "fixing" "relieving" or "dealing with" a crisis that, in reality, was temporary. We may have felt like things were fixed until... they broke. Once some of these really nasty wounds began to surface, we could no longer deny that we'd been through a life-altering experience which was now taking a toll on our current lives.

Beloved, when you start with abortion healing, it places you on the path towards overall healing. Healing is a process, a multi-step, multi-layered journey of getting pulled out of the muck and mire. Heal in one area and you will often find a domino effect occurring as the healing tools help you to heal other trauma(s) in your life. Stay with the process.

BIBLE CONNECTION: Consider the story of Sarai, wife of Abram. She took it upon herself to help God fulfill His promise to give them children (Genesis 16 and 18). The birth of Ishmael caused Sarai to feel humiliated and "less than" in comparison to Hagar her maid and Ishmaels' mom. Instead of recognizing her part in the fiasco, Sarai took out her woundedness on Abram and Hagar. She stayed stuck in the muck she created and blamed everyone else for the consequences. REFLECTION: Sometimes, when we sin, we fail to recognize that our poor decisions caused self-inflicted wounds. Be patient, follow God's plan when it comes to reproduction and avoid the wound.

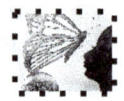

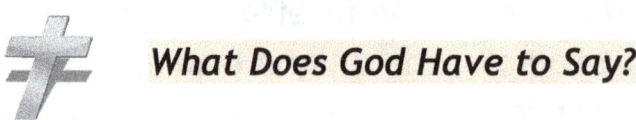 What Does God Have to Say?

8 and the two are united into one.' Since they are no longer two but one, 9 let no one split apart what God has joined together."
Mark 10:8-9

God originally intended sexual intercourse to join two people together throughout their earthly lives, in a binding covenant agreement. Unfortunately, sex has become a casual event for most Americans because we treat it as an animal *act* without physical, emotional or spiritual consequences. Without the covenant of marriage, our sinful desires for sex tend to rule over our ability to remain abstinent. Physical intimacy before marriage has become our new normal and "why buy the cow if you can get the milk for free" is our mantra. Cohabitation is now culturally supported over marriage. God's intention for us was marriage and then sex, in that order. That statement may sound "old fashioned" to some yet God's plan for our lives hasn't changed. When we impatiently change His plans for marriage and sex we suffer multiple lasting consequences.

- What do you remember being taught about the intimate bonds of sexual intercourse, if anything?

- When we have sex there is chemical bonding that occurs. Watch this five minute video on sexual bonding, Oxytocin: the Big Deal About Sex and then share your thoughts.

- Was the father of your child(ren) your first sexual partner? Was the arrangement consensual or coerced?

- Did the possibility of becoming pregnant cross your mind(s)?

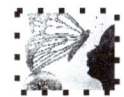

- Does your baby's father have other children? If so, how does that make you feel?

You made all the delicate, inner parts of my body and knit me together in my mother's womb.
Psalm 139:13

- How did you feel when you first found out you were pregnant?

- What was the response of the baby's father?

- Did the fathers' response influence your choice(s) to abort?

- If you told your mom (or other female confidant), what was her response?

- Did your mom's response influence your choice(s) to abort?

- Who did you choose to tell? Who did you leave in the dark?

- What did the clinic say about your baby's development at the time of your abortion? In other words, were you told how many weeks old your baby was? Were you given an ultrasound?

PLEASE TAKE A DEEP BREATH BEFORE OPENING THE LINK BELOW. THE LINK WILL TAKE YOU TO PHOTOS OF ACRYLIC BABIES AGES 8 TO 12 WEEKS. Be aware that the majority of abortions occur during these gestational weeks, but that yours may have been outside of these timeframes. Breathe through it without self-judgment.

[First Trimester Baby Models](#)

- How did seeing the baby models make you feel?

- What surprised you most about the development of your child(ren) after seeing the baby models?

- Were you given any details about the age and development of your baby at the abortion clinic either in print or verbally?

Let us take a look at God's creation in time lapse video form from [LiveAction and Baby Olivia.](#)

[Click here to watch a live gentle birth](#). (Please treat this video as optional and save it for another time as guided).

My wounds fester and stink because of my foolish sins. I am bent over and racked with pain. All day long I walk around filled with grief. A raging fever burns within me, and my health is broken. I am exhausted and completely crushed. My groans come from an anguished heart.
Psalm 38:5-8

- Now that you have had a minute to think about it, if your abortion were a wound, how would you describe it? Be as descriptive as you need to be. You may paint a word picture or use drawings. Take your time.

- What was your opinion about abortion prior to becoming pregnant?

- How did the idea of your having the abortion(s) come about? Who brought it up and how did the plan proceed?

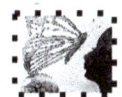

- Was your abortion advised by your doctor or the clinic personnel? Did you feel as if you had a choice to change your mind?

- Take some time to detail the abortion(s). Whether it was a surgical procedure(s) or the abortion pills, write out as many details as you can in a separate and secure area.

Be gentle with yourself as many images may come back or specifics may or may not be hidden from your conscious mind for now. Include ages and dates as they come back. Be sure to reach out to a counselor, prayer warrior or trusted friend during this time. Some images may appear in dreams or as repressed memories. Write as much down as you can even if it appears confusing as this will help you to release.

Is there no medicine in Gilead? Is there no physician there? Why is there no healing for the wounds of my people?
Jeremiah 8:22

- Did you suffer any unexpected side effects from the abortion pills or the procedure? Where did you go for treatment for complications? (There is an organization called Operation Outcry that collects testimonies about abortion facilities that you can contact if you want to register a complaint).

- After the abortion(s), to whom did you go for comfort?

- Did the 'Strong Black Woman' idea kick in to help you get through the abortion? If yes, how was it demonstrated to others?

- What was your relationship with the father of your child(ren) like afterwards?

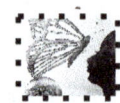

- What was the after care support like from the clinic responsible for the abortion?

- Were you conscious of using anything specific such as alcohol, drugs, overeating or sex etc. to dull the post abortion pain?

Then your salvation will come like the dawn, and your wounds will quickly heal. Your godliness will lead you forward, and the glory of the LORD will protect you from behind.
Isaiah 58:8

- How did you hear about *abortion healing* or *abortion recovery*?

- What were some of your reservations about getting involved with an abortion recovery program?

- What length of time was it between hearing about an abortion recovery program and your connecting with one?

- Had you heard of or known anything about pregnancy resource centers prior to or when you were pregnant?

- What is your sense of God's presence in the healing process up till now?

He heals the brokenhearted and bandages their wounds.
Psalm 147:3

- In what area(s) did you feel the most broken? Was it your relationship with God, the baby's father, your parents, yourself, etc.? Write each broken relationship on a post-it note or index card.

Check In: (click to do a Guided Tension Release from Head to Toe).

Expert Opinion

- "The Benefits of Trauma Healing" by Dr. Joy DeGruy-54 minutes.
- "Brokenness" by Voddie Baucham-54 minutes

Let's share our stories around a previous healing journey or a time when you felt like you made it through an emotional crisis.

- How did telling your story make you feel?

- How could you relate to your sister's story?

- How might you apply previous healing tools to your abortion healing?

Full Circle Moment of Reflection

Be still for a moment and reflect on what you have heard, read and experienced thus far. Feel free to share your letter written to your younger self and your photo with the group. You may also consider sharing what you've written with another trusted person if you are working on this alone. Don't forget to journal about what comes to your attention.

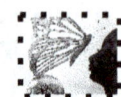

Sylvia Blakely

Arise, And Fly Free!

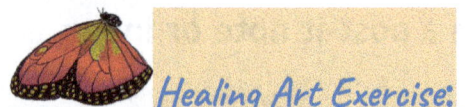

Healing Art Exercise: "Now and Later"

Using our butterfly, we will explore the transitional process and growth that comes from healing. Click on the image for detailed instructions on CANVA to help you complete the exercise.

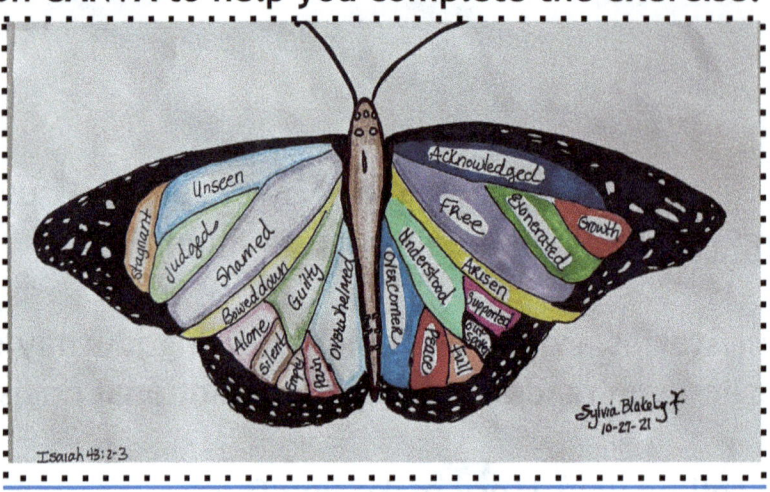

Notes:

www.AriseArtists.com   @arisedaughterfl   AriseDaughter@gmail.com

Sylvia Blakely 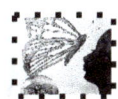 Arise, And Fly Free!

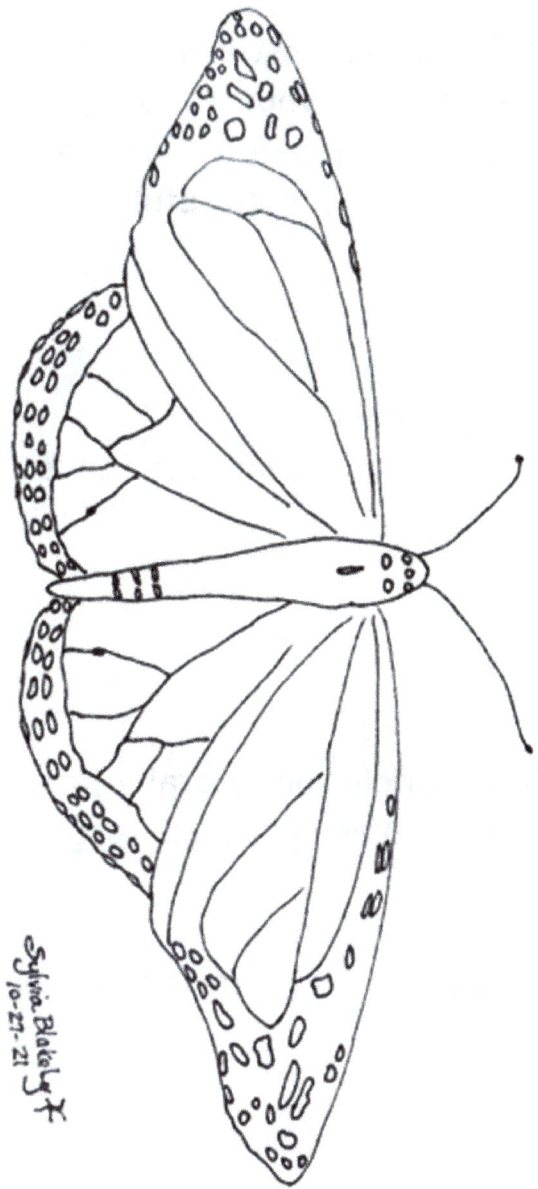

Printable Template by Sylvia Blakely

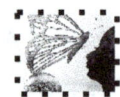

Write Your Prayer

Assemble the broken relationship post-it notes or index cards you completed earlier and ask God, in your written prayer, to help you mend them. Include a name for God or a characteristic of God in your prayer. Include three things you are grateful for.

Songs

- *"Prodigal Son"* by Fred Hammond.
- *"Deliver Me (This is My Exodus)"* by Donald Lawrence.

Homework

1. Read the three brief articles on "Moral Injury Through a Biblical Lens" written by Sylvia Blakely RN, MS: Article 1; Article 2 and Article 3.

2. Visit the virtual Wellness Basket in Canva.

Notes:

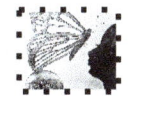

Chapter 4

Understanding Our Pain

"If you are silent about your pain, they'll kill you and say you enjoyed it."
Zora Neale Hurston

Pain is not new to us as a people. Our collective pain, caused by generational trauma, is something we are just now beginning to acknowledge even when society at large doesn't want us to. How do we reconcile that the harm that was done to us for generations contributed to the harm that we caused? Not recognizing our pain is what has kept this country from the deep healing that needs to occur. It is time to look at our pain as a nation in order to heal from the generational trauma that has led to a culture of abortion (we promise to tackle that healing conversation in another curriculum).

Healing of any sort is tedious. Healing is hard work and has repercussions even when it is done well. We have learned through prior painful experiences that there are physical, emotional and psychological wounds that seem to get worse every time we attempt to heal. The clean up of the persistent wounds is often left up to the person(s) who has suffered the most; that may not seem fair but it is often true. We sometimes want to give in, go the easy route and just *"let it be."* But letting the past go is not the same thing as embracing the change that the past causes. Each of us experiences a psychological change after significant personal or national events. The legalization of abortion and the trauma that haunts us is a nationally significant event that we have not acknowledged. Our tendency to "double down" by justifying and legalizing abortion has created some of the most convoluted and disturbing arguments for abortion heard yet. However, God is not mocked!

Our Judeo-Christian ethic says that we are "Imago Dei" or made in the image of God. We also believe in the commandment that "You shall not murder." (Exodus 20:13). What slavery did was to destroy the soul of a nation by killing its moral foundation. As Christians, we have been taught to believe that life is sacred and to be protected and yet, we have allowed our legal system to condone the willful taking of an innocent person's life up until birth. This is how slavery and abortion are intimately connected: We need to acknowledge that the morality of the nation was debased when people were allowed to be categorized and treated as less than human. Names such as "savage" and "monkey" easily gave rise to "blob of tissue" and "clump of cells." The terminology meant to confuse us about the sanctity of life allowed humans to manipulate and denigrate other humans. By using terms such as "fetus" or "product of conception," the abortion industry further worked to dehumanize our children despite undisputed scientific opinion that life begins at conception (read the article, "The Facts and Doubts About Beginning of the Human Life and Personality.").

Once we decided that the life we were taking was less than human or that the new life was a threat in some way, then we could justify our choice to end it. And yet, by agreeing to the destruction of a person that was not guilty of anything in particular, we struggle now with the unveiled fact that our abortion went against, not only our personal moral code but God's.

None of this is easy to write, nor is it easy to read and acknowledge. For us to move forward with our healing from our abortion(s), we will have to stand in the tense gap of knowing that what we have done was immoral and wrong. This is also when we will begin to accept the negative effect(s) that decision has had on our physical and psychological lives as well as the lives of others. It is this burden that we have to bear in order to turn the tide of personal opinion regarding the worth of human life. Regardless of the situation or circumstance, we will only bear our share of the responsibility if we can acknowledge the pain we have experienced and the pain we have caused.

The phenomenon known as *moral injury* describes the wounded psyche of a person after they make a decision that goes against their personal moral code. The concept of moral injury has been extensively studied in military personnel. For example, it has been reported by researchers that moral injury causes guilt, trauma, and depression when a direct military order contradicts a soldier's moral code. If left unacknowledged and untreated, moral injury can lead to suicidal thoughts and, in some cases attempts at or completion of a suicidal act. *(If you or someone you know is having suicidal thoughts, please dial 988 to talk or text).*

Before a service man or woman is placed in a position to end a person's life in a combat situation, they have to believe that the person deserved to die. The service person was probably told that the "offender" had done something evil or was threatening the lives of others. During wartime training, soldiers are typically subjected to propaganda designed to dehumanize the enemy. This training allows the conscious mind the justification to take the life of someone they do not know. If a particular person or people group died but are later found to be innocent or blameless, the service person is left feeling morally damaged because of the lingering guilt and shame about their actions.

Through the above example, we can begin to see how our abortion(s) morally injured us.   We believed the propaganda that our baby was "nothing," a "blob of cells," not "viable" or not a distinct "person."   We also believed that abortion was "health care" and we took the life of someone innocent because of false beliefs. By doing the opposite of caring for our baby, we are now faced with the moral injury our choice has caused.

How do we begin the moral healing process ? We can start with following the example of King David in Psalm 51 NLT:

1. Naming the event and those involved.
2. Repenting to the one we've grieved the most (God) and asking for forgiveness.
3. Sharing our story with someone in a healing community we trust so that no one feels alone.
4. Grieving our loss(es)
5. Forgiving all who harmed us and taking responsibility for those we have harmed.
6. Giving proper acknowledgement of our child/children through a memorial service.
7. Learning how to speak up for life in our circles of influence such as within our family.

Now that we have acknowledged our loss(es) and their effects on us, how do we live with all that has happened? As we have seen, our past greatly informs our present and sometimes directs our future. There have been many societal factors that contributed to our abortion(s) and some of them were out of our control. There may also have been other circumstances surrounding our abortion(s) that we have yet to really explore. Many women (and some men) feel manipulation was used to force a decision for abortion. The coercion could have come from their partner, either sets of grandparents, trusted friends or even clergy.

Can you identify the many people or entities involved in your abortion decision? Take a few minutes to name each person. Use the

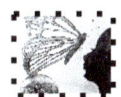

pie chart below to assign a slice of the pie to the people involved. Try to estimate how much of the pie they were responsible for. Take your time and be sure not to assign 100% of the pie to yourself.

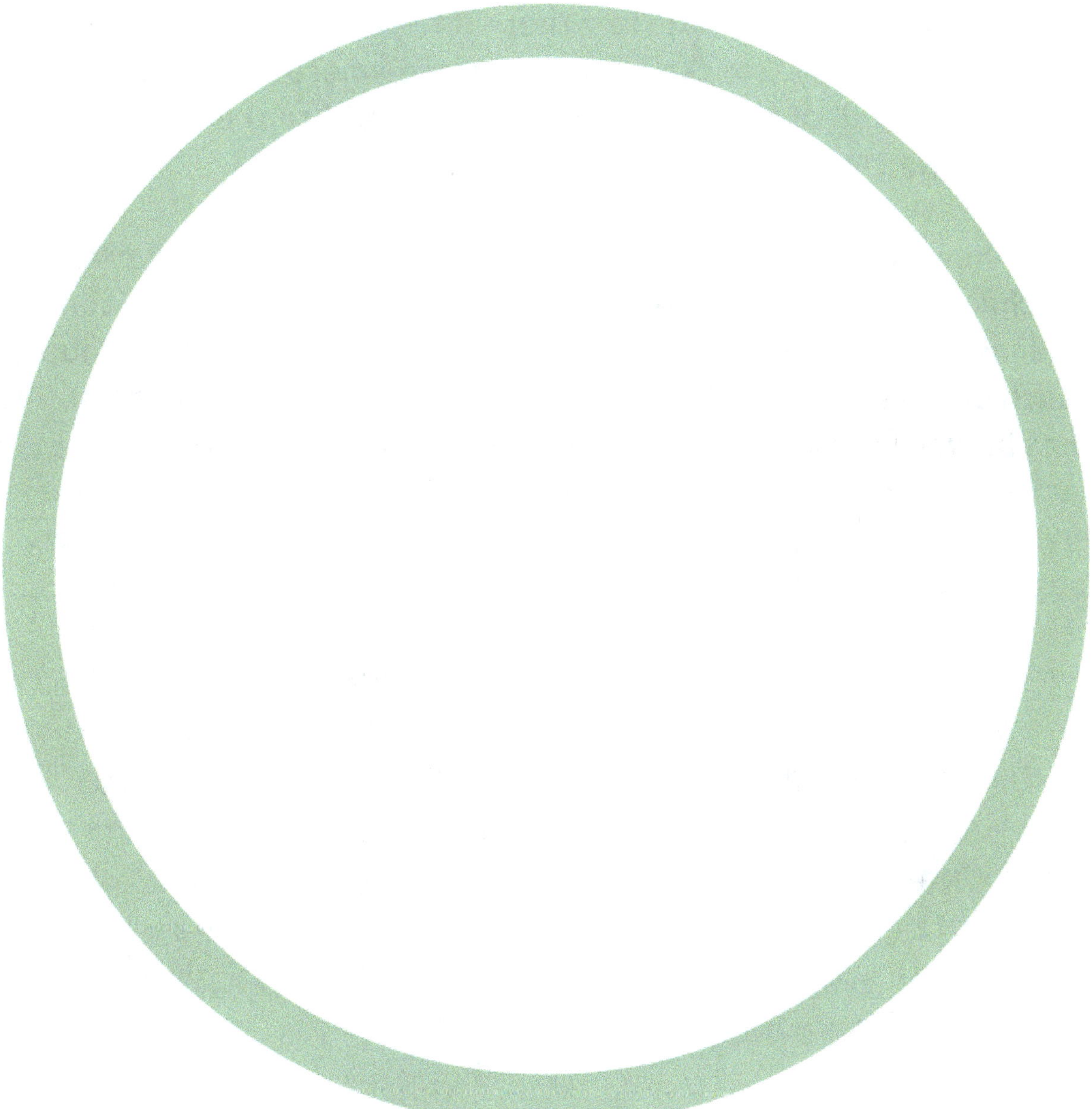

Printable Template Sourced from Google images

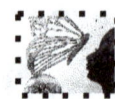

Part of the healing walk this week involved acknowledging the pain of our abortion(s) as well as the contributions made from society, family etc. Doing the work of assigning responsibility to ourselves and others for our abortion(s) might at first appear to be the same as assigning blame. That's OK; start there if necessary. Once we look at the situation clearly, we can come to a place where we can properly see our part in all of this and grieve our lost child(ren) in humility and true repentance.

Whew! This chapter was a lot. But know this: you are a *breacher*. *Breacher* is a military term roughly meaning "first in." In this context it means you are the one willing to be the first in your family group to breach or burst through the door of healing from your abortion(s). It takes bravery to complete the *mission* of reconciliation with our gracious heavenly Father. The healing work you are doing will have generational consequences by interrupting old patterns of behavior. Congratulations, keep your head down and keep moving forward!

<u>Bible connection</u>: Consider the story of David and Bathsheba in 2 Samuel chapters 11 and 12. Davids' sins were many, from lust to adultery to murder. David crafted elaborate schemes to make his sins appear acceptable. This "man after God's own heart" went against the moral code of God and himself. When the prophet Nathan called David out so that he could face his sins he immediately recognized his wrongs and repented. Nathan was a gift from God sent to change a heart going in the wrong direction. It was a year later that he wrote his famous lament in Psalm 51 where he recognized his brokenness. <u>Reflection</u>: When we wound God, God has to wound us through Holy Spirit conviction in order to heal us. The healing process is a gift from God; trust God and take advantage of the promise of reconciliation He has for all of His people.

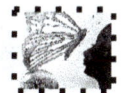

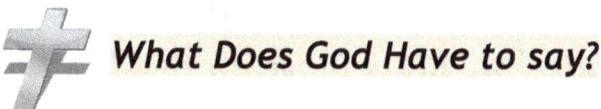 **What Does God Have to say?**

If anyone takes a human life, that person's life will also be taken by human hands. For God made human beings in his own image.
Genesis 9:6

- Why was God's warning against bloodshed so severe?

- In what ways did we place ourselves on the same moral level as God?

- Why was "an eye for an eye," the legal code?

37 They even sacrificed their sons and their daughters to the demons. 38 They shed innocent blood, the blood of their sons and daughters. By sacrificing them to the idols of Canaan, they polluted the land with murder. 39 They defiled themselves by their evil deeds, and their love of idols was adultery in the LORD's sight. 40 That is why the LORD's anger burned against his people, and he abhorred his own special possession.
Psalm 106:37-40

- What is the difference between what is legal and what is moral?

- Prior to your abortion, would you have considered it child sacrifice? If no, why not? If yes, why?

- Why must God separate Himself from the sins of His people?

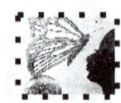

16 There are six things the LORD hates--no, seven things he detests: 17 haughty eyes, a lying tongue, hands that kill the innocent, 18 a heart that plots evil, feet that race to do wrong, 19 a false witness who pours out lies, a person who sows discord in a family.

Proverbs 6:16-19

- Using the above verses as a springboard, how might you describe your behavior in regards to your abortion(s)? For example, might you have *proudly* stood up for the *right* to an abortion? Carefully go down the list of offenses to God (proud look, lying tongue, etc.) and describe in detail how your thoughts or actions matched up. (Please keep in mind that we are not judging ourselves; we are simply being transparent and stating our feelings.)

Read the story of Joseph in Genesis 37:18-36 and how his brothers sold him into captivity. Recall what the eldest brother, Reuben, said to his other brothers in Genesis 42:22 *"Didn't I tell you not to sin against the boy?" Reuben asked. "But you wouldn't listen. And now we have to answer for his blood!"*

- Was there anyone or any institution in your life at that time that told you abortion was wrong?

- What were the reasons you gave at the time to continue? (If the abortion was forced then you may skip this question.)

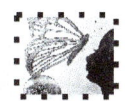

5 The LORD observed the extent of human wickedness on the earth, and he saw that everything they thought or imagined was consistently and totally evil. 6 So the LORD was sorry he had ever made them and put them on the earth. It broke his heart.
Genesis 6:5-6

- Were you aware before the abortion(s) that God's heart could be grieved? How did you come to know this?

- What punishment did you think you deserved for the abortion(s)?

For no person will be justified [freed of guilt and declared righteous] in His sight by [trying to do] the works of the Law. For through the Law we become conscious of sin [and the recognition of sin directs us toward repentance, but provides no remedy for sin]."
Romans 3:20 AMP

- How long did you try to do *righteous works* to *make it right* with God?

- What were some of your *righteous works*?

Then they cried out to the LORD in their trouble, and He saved them from their distresses. He sent His word and healed them, and rescued them from their destruction. Let them give thanks to the LORD for His lovingkindness, and for His wonderful acts to the children of men!
Psalm 107:19-21 AMP

- How would you describe your *cry out to the Lord*?

- What have you learned so far from the Word of God that is helping you to heal?

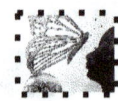

- What does being saved from destruction mean for you?

13 Are any of you suffering hardships? You should pray. Are any of you happy? You should sing praises. 14 Are any of you sick? You should call for the elders of the church to come and pray over you, anointing you with oil in the name of the Lord. 15 Such a prayer offered in faith will heal the sick, and the Lord will make you well. And if you have committed any sins, you will be forgiven. 16 Confess your sins to each other and pray for each other so that you may be healed. The earnest prayer of a righteous person has great power and produces wonderful results.

James 5:13-16

- Confession (not righteous works!) is the first step in accepting responsibility for our abortion(s). How difficult has it been to share your guilt and shame with others? How about with God?

- Have you come to a place of regret for the abortion(s)? If so, how might you confess and express your regret to God? To your child(ren)? Let us take time to write a letter of regret and repentance to God.

But God showed his great love for us by sending Christ to die for us while we were still sinners.

Romans 5:8

- Did it cross your mind that Christ came to sacrifice His life for the sin of abortion?

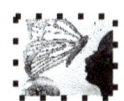

- Do you believe in your heart that the blood of Christ covers the sin of your abortion(s)? If yes, why? If no, why not?

And not only [that], but we also rejoice in God through our Lord Jesus Christ, through whom we have now received the reconciliation.
Romans 5:11 NKJV

- What is the biblical definition of *reconciliation*?

- Our Father sees you through the lens of His Son Jesus and the blood He shed. Have you been able to accept this truth?

15 This is a trustworthy saying, and everyone should accept it: "Christ Jesus came into the world to save sinners"--and I am the worst of them all.
1 Timothy 1:15

- How long have you believed you were the *WORST* sinner and therefore beyond saving?

- Who else among God's elect can claim that title? (Bible figures David, Moses, Paul etc. can add some context).

The Lord wants to refresh you through the gift of Holy Spirit: As it says in Acts 3:19 *Now repent of your sins and turn to God, so that your sins may be wiped away.* Describe one way that you can come before the presence of the Lord to be refreshed.

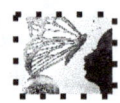

If you confess with your mouth that Jesus is Lord and believe in your heart that God raised him from the dead, you will be saved.
Romans 10:9

If you have not yet received the Lord Jesus Christ into your heart, may this be the hour? You can accept the Lord into your heart and life whether you are doing this study alone or in a group. If you believe in your heart and confess with your mouth that Jesus Christ is God's Son, that He came to repair our relationship with God the Father, that He was crucified for our sins, that He rose from the dead and now sits at the right hand of the Father actively interceding for you, then you are saved!

Pray this prayer when you are ready:

Father, I admit that I have sinned and am a sinner. I've been trying to take control of life decisions that belong to you and I am so sorry. I believe You sent Your Son to sacrifice Himself to blot out my many sins including my abortion(s). I believe that Jesus rose from the dead and is interceding on my behalf. I accept Jesus as my Lord, Savior and King, and I commit myself to serving You through His example now and in the days ahead. In Jesus's precious and mighty name I pray.

Amen.

This can also be a prayer of rededication

Acts 2:38 says, *Peter replied, "Each of you must repent of your sins and turn to God, and be baptized in the name of Jesus Christ for the forgiveness of your sins. Then you will receive the gift of the Holy Spirit.*

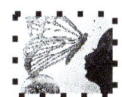

If you are working on this study alone and have never been baptized and would like to be, please contact Sylvia Blakely at arisedaughter@gmail.com. For those of you who have a facilitator, you can ask her for more information on how a local church can assist you with being baptized. Connecting with like-minded Christians who can hear your story and support your growth will be crucial in the days ahead.

<u>*Baptism and Discipleship plans:*</u>

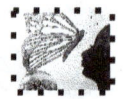

==Check In==: "Praise Break."
Take a few moments to give God praise in any way you would like. (You may go off camera at this time.)

==Expert Opinion==

- Read: "What is Moral Injury?" by Syracuse University.

Let's hear Sister Sylvia's Story. as someone who has walked through the steps of accepting her pain.

I was a junior in college and had been dating and having sex with the same person since freshman year. As we began to grow apart I knew he wouldn't be the person I would eventually marry. We had sex one more time before our breakup and to both of our surprises, the condom broke. This was towards the end of the school year and I was getting set to go home and work for the summer. I began to notice my breasts were tender and I was sleeping and urinating a lot. As a nursing student I quickly figured out I might be pregnant. I picked up the phone and frantically made two calls: one to the father of the baby to let him know about the pregnancy and my desire to have an abortion and one to my middle sister whom I knew could help me arrange the "procedure." Both of them offered financial assistance of some sort; I remember it was around $250. I did not tell my parents I wasn't coming home until everything was arranged and then I only shared that I was going to hang out with my sister for the summer. I was afraid of messing up my "good girl" reputation and of putting my school scholarship in jeopardy so, I kept everything a secret. I was also fairly certain that my parents wouldn't have been supportive of an out-of-wedlock child since I knew my oldest sister was made to give up her first child for adoption at 16. I took the bus to Ann Arbor, Michigan and shortly set up the abortion at the Planned Parenthood clinic. I don't remember everything about that day but I do remember not wanting to look around at the other women in the room. I was taken back to a small locker room and told to disrobe. I was given a pill and a dixie cup full of water to drink as I waited. I then remember being directed into a very large, very cold room and helped onto a hard exam table. The doctor came in and turned on a machine that sounded horrible. He never looked at me or addressed me before or after the "procedure." I remember the nurse holding my hand and locking eyes with me. I squeezed so hard once the pain and pressure hit me that I'm sure I hurt her but she kept her gaze steady and kind. I quickly glanced over at the canister attached to the machine and I could see blood and white flecks of tissue; at that point my mind went blank. Afterwards, the nurse helped me up and took me to a rather large waiting room with other women who looked as dazed and confused as I was. I remember being offered some crackers and juice and shortly after, I got dressed and went to my sister's apartment. I remember sleeping the day away ignoring the physical and emotional pain I was feeling. I stayed with her the rest of the summer and immediately got into a relationship that I really didn't want. I returned to school in the fall and behaved like nothing ever happened. I wore the mask of denial for 20 years. The only person I chose to share my abortion with decades later was my then serious boyfriend who became my fiance' and husband.

- How did this story make you feel?

- How could you relate to the difficult situation?

- What moral convictions have changed for you since your abortion?

Full Circle Moment of Reflection

Be still for a moment and reflect on what you have heard, read and experienced thus far. Feel free to share any comments on the homework regarding moral injury. Take time to journal what this chapter has brought up for you.

Healing Art Exercise: "The Mask"

Through this exercise, we will take a look at all of the conflicting emotions within us, what we choose to share and what we choose to hide. Click on the image for instructions in CANVA.

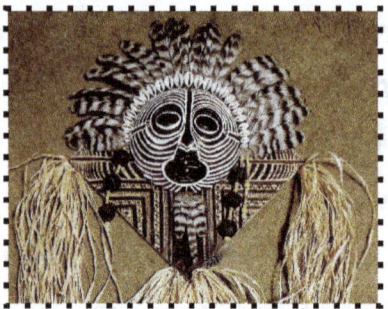

Notes:

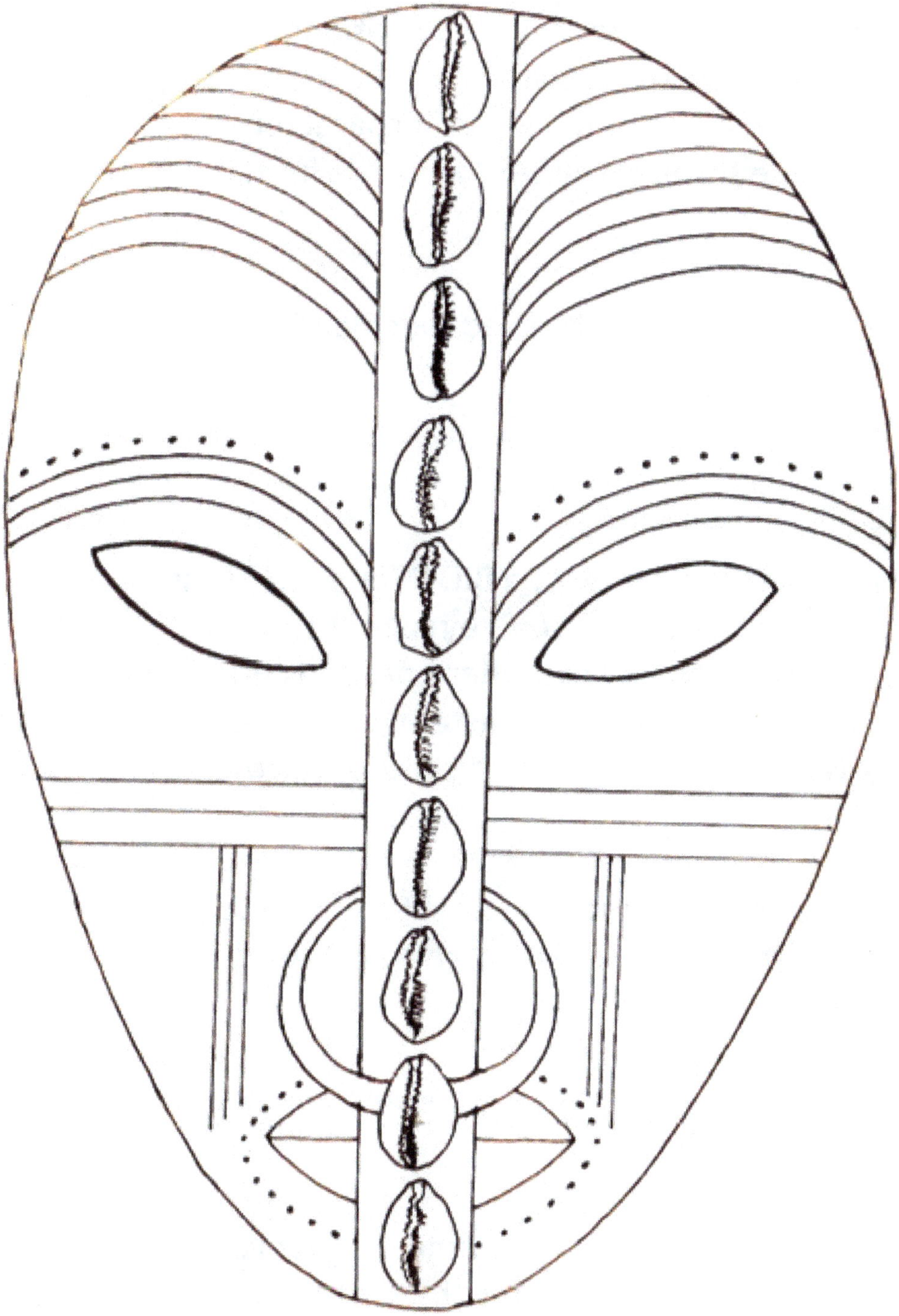

Sylvia Blakely 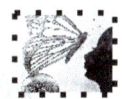 Arise, And Fly Free!

Printable Template by Freda Abbott-Ayodele

www.AriseArtists.com @arisedaughterfl AriseDaughter@gmail.com

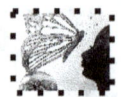

Write Your Prayer

Write a prayer of thanksgiving for salvation or a prayer of thanksgiving for reconciliation; write whichever prayer applies to you. Include one of the names of God or a characteristic of God in your prayer. Include three things you are grateful for.

Songs

- "Breathe Into Me Oh Lord" by Fred Hammond.
- "Lord, Make Me Over" by Tonex.

Homework: "Halfway Hallelujah"

Sis, let's take a breath… a BIG DEEP BREATH and acknowledge from whence we've come! You've made it through the first half of the study. It's time to give praise where praise is due and that is to our almighty Father. It wasn't easy listening to His gentle words and following His prompts to get to this place, so rejoice and give God the glory.

Consider this another unique moment for a *Praise Break*. Feel how you feel, and in the midst, again, give God the glory! Here are a couple of songs to praise with:

- "I'm In The Midst Of It All" by Fred Hammond and United Tenors.
- "In the Middle" by Isaac Carree.

DEFINITELY consider this a time of celebration if you've accepted Jesus as your Lord and Savior for the first time! Know that all of Heaven is rejoicing with you!

Check in with your Wellness Plan. Is it accomplishing the goal or does it need some adjustment?

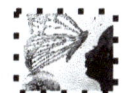

Journal your pent up emotions or feelings about moving forward. HOMEWORK: What would you say to your bestie if she said, "This is too hard!!" What words of encouragement or Bible verses could you pour over her? Write her a letter.

Begin to think about how you would like to remember your child(ren) at our memorial service…

Let's continue, ladies!

Notes:

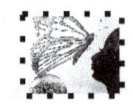

Chapter 5

Dealing With The Anger

"You should be angry. You must not be bitter. Bitterness is like cancer. It eats upon the host. It doesn't do anything to the object of its displeasure."
Maya Angelou

There is a great work of repentance that must happen on a national level in order for God to heal our land from the stain of abortion. For starters, we must acknowledge that the horror of almost 370 years of slavery and Jim Crow is at the root of abortion in America. The history surrounding enslavers manipulating Black women's child-bearing ability is at the root of abortion. Our history of forced breeding, commodification and later sterilization of black and brown bodies must be studied and faced head on to understand how abortion was legalized. Abortion has deep deep roots and we must be diligent to dig all of them up if we want to reject the modern notion that, "Abortion is Normal." Nothing that happened to us as black women in this country was normal.

This would be an appropriate time to pause in remembrance of those deeply harmed, including you...

America was founded on an ungodly disdain for anyone other than those who were the colonizers. All men are created equal in the eyes of the Lord but, all men certainly were not treated equally no matter what the constitution of this nation states. Through unjust laws and unfair practices, African-American and First Nations people have borne the brunt of unfair treatment in this country. When a people group exercises unbridled injustice against others, hubris can follow. With hubris came a tendency for the colonizers to believe that they were gods and that they had the right to manipulate life as they saw fit.

God is not mocked and He will not tolerate anyone setting His precepts aside (Galatians 6:7). It was not God's intended purpose for anyone to take life and death into their own hands. As image bearers of the Creator Himself, each human being that has ever been conceived has a purpose and plan for their life that God alone determines. God doesn't have to explain His purposes to man and we don't have to understand them (Ecclesiastes 11:5 AMP). God is a God of justice and righteousness: Violate His plans and you fundamentally hurt the heart of God.

Thankfully, we serve a God that is *slow to anger and ready to "relent [His sentence of] evil [when His people genuinely repent]?"* (Joel 2:13b AMP). God says in 2 Chronicles 7:14 *Then if my people who are called by my name will humble themselves and pray and seek my face and turn from their wicked ways, I will hear from heaven and will forgive their sins and restore their land.*

Humility and repentance come before forgiveness, and forgiveness of sins is a gift from God. Our way back to God was established by Him a long time ago. Two questions remain then: is the nation willing to do what it takes to be reconciled to God? And do we, as post-abortive black women, need to wait until the nation is reconciled to God before we ourselves are reconciled? We can pause to reflect on that...

Our anger at how we have been mistreated in this country is justified, but rarely discussed. Internalized anger, however, is an important topic to examine especially in relation to our physical, emotional and spiritual health. The negative effects of anger on our well being is now an established fact. The quality and quantity of our lives are being adversely affected by systemic racism. Overt racist policies, the microaggressions of everyday life, and the flagrant disregard for our culture and feelings, is enough to make us put on an armor of "vigilant anger." The hostile environment we live in has caused us to be constantly bombarded by stress hormones, such as cortisol and testosterone. Cortisol can cause harmful inflammatory responses in the body and influence the development of chronic illnesses such as hypertension and a depressed immune system. (Read this article from Mayo Clinic). Cortisol is also a key player in our "fight or flight" survival response system. When we perceive a threat to our personhood we may easily become conditioned to either fight or flee the situation. Many of us have experienced the often overwhelming feeling of wanting to punch someone that has emotionally hurt us and yet we've kept that response in check. Feeling like we have to defend ourselves most of our work day can be very taxing to our overall health especially if outstanding feelings are left unresolved. Where do you offload all of that? Unfortunately, we pour out our unresolved emotions onto loved ones including ourselves.

Let's key in for a moment on *anger* since it is so harmful. Anger is actually considered a secondary emotion or the manifestation of other deeper emotions such as grief, fear, unresolved anxiety, sadness, broken trust, etc. (Healthypsych.com). Anger can also be triggered when you sense disrespect for your personhood. Be honest: Have you ever felt like this is one emotion that you have the right to protect yourself with? The caricature of the "Angry Black Woman" has many understandable and justifiable roots. Who else has had to endure what we have and still be expected to stay sane, sweet, godly *and* strong? We can be seen as angry on the outside all while crumbling on the inside.

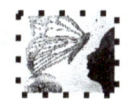

We have to acknowledge that some foundational work is needed to repair our grieving, angry broken hearts. Undoing years, sometimes decades, of damage is going to take time. God's Word and the intervention of Holy Spirit is our path out of darkness and into the marvelous light. We have to rely on Jesus as our example to set us free from the bondage of anger because He is the Way, the Truth and the Life ([John 14:6](#)). My sisters, we have been bound so long by grief, fear, anxiety, stress, trauma etc. that we can't see how restrictive the armor of anger has been. Don't you want to get back the days that anger, frustration, depression, numbness and unforgiveness have taken from you? How long have you been shackled to your emotions and unable to move forward in freedom?

Let's take a moment to name all the people and institutions you feel anger towards regarding your abortion(s). It might include anyone you hold responsible or accountable for your abortion(s) in this or in past generations. Don't hold back! Start where you want to start Sis, and let it go wherever it goes.

At some point in our healing journey it will be crucial to acknowledge this deeper point: that the anger we turned towards ourselves has been a destructive force to our soul. The guilt and shame we carry because of our abortion(s) has been like extra weights on already manicled feet. Know this: God wants us fully healed and truly free.

Even the righteous anger we hold must be tempered to be used correctly. Be realistic and sincere; If anger has been your weapon of choice for years, it will be difficult to lay it down. Being able to forgive those who hurt you (even if it is a whole nation) may seem impossible. But we serve a God who has been through all that we have been through and more. He understands being unjustly treated. He bore the weight of our guilt and shame and He is willing to forgive it all. Jesus is our true example of how to forgive what seems unforgivable.

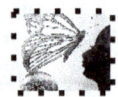

Even on the cross, Jesus gave us the model of how to forgive everybody. It's only through God that all things are possible!

BIBLE CONNECTION: CONSIDER THE STORY OF KING SAUL'S DAUGHTER AND DAVID'S FIRST WIFE MICHAL IN FIRST AND SECOND SAMUEL. IF ANYONE HAD A "RIGHT" TO BE ANGRY ABOUT HOW HER LIFE TURNED OUT IT WAS MICHAL. SHE WAS USED AS A POLITICAL PAWN AND TREATED LIKE A POSSESSION FOR MUCH OF HER LIFE. THERE ALWAYS SEEMED TO BE CONDITIONS PLACED AROUND HER WORTH BY THE MEN IN HER LIFE. HER LOVE FOR DAVID MORPHED INTO CONTEMPT AS THE YEARS PASSED. WHEN SHE FINALLY ARRIVED AT THE PLACE WHERE SHE SHOULD HAVE BEEN SECURE AS THE WIFE OF THE MOST POWERFUL MAN IN THE KINGDOM, SHE ALLOWED ANGER AND BITTERNESS TO CURSE HER HUSBAND AND KING. INSTEAD OF REJOICING IN THE POWER OF THE GOD WHO RESTORED HER POSITION SHE ALLOWED UNFORGIVENESS TO DIG BITTER ROOTS. AS A RESULT, THE LORD CLOSED MICHAL'S WOMB AND SHE NEVER BORE DAVID ANY CHILDREN. SHE FORFEITED HER PLACE IN THE LINEAGE OF KINGS GOD PROMISED HER HUSBAND.
REFLECTION: BEING BITTER DOES NOT MAKE YOU BETTER. LIKE MICHAL, OUR BEGINNING MAY HAVE BEEN ROUGH BUT GOD HAS BETTER PLANS FOR OUR FUTURE WHEN WE TRUST IN HIM TO DIG OUT OUR BITTER ROOTS BEFORE THEY POISON US AND OUR FUTURE.

 *What Does God Have to Say?*

In Romans 12:1-2 (AMP), it states, *"Therefore I urge you, brothers and sisters, by the mercies of God, to present your bodies [dedicating all of yourselves, set apart] as a living sacrifice, holy and well-pleasing to God, which is your rational (logical, intelligent) act of worship. And do not be conformed to this world [any longer with its superficial values and customs], but be transformed and progressively changed [as you mature spiritually] by the renewing of your mind [focusing on godly values and ethical attitudes], so that you may prove [for yourselves] what the will of God is, that which is good and acceptable and perfect [in His plan and purpose for you]."*

- Why is Paul *urging* his brothers and sisters towards change?

- Why does it take the *mercies of God* to do the work necessary to change?

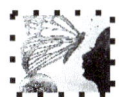

- Is our unresolved anger *well-pleasing* to God? Why or why not?

- What will it mean for you to unconform from the worldly view of anger? Take some time and get detailed. Include both thoughts and actions which stem from the heart.

And Jesus entered the temple [grounds] and drove out [with force] all who were buying and selling [birds and animals for sacrifice] in the temple area, and He turned over the tables of the moneychangers [who made a profit exchanging foreign money for temple coinage] and the chairs of those who were selling doves [for sacrifice]. Jesus said to them, "It is written [in Scripture], 'MY HOUSE SHALL BE CALLED A HOUSE OF PRAYER'; but you are making it a ROBBERS' DEN.
Matthew 21:12-13 AMP

- How was Jesus' anger righteous and how did He avoid sin in this situation?

- Do we have a right to *righteous anger* and how can it be directed effectively?

BE ANGRY [at sin--at immorality, at injustice, at ungodly behavior], YET DO NOT SIN; do not let your anger [cause you shame, nor allow it to] last until the sun goes down. And do not give the devil an opportunity [to lead you into sin by holding a grudge, or nurturing anger, or harboring resentment, or cultivating bitterness].
Ephesians 4:26-27 AMP

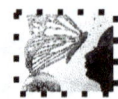

- Why does God allow anger but not sinning while angry?

- What injustice, immorality and ungodly behavior have you encountered that makes you angry?

'Vengeance is Mine, and retribution, In due time their foot will slip; For the day of their disaster is at hand, And their doom hurries to meet them.'
Deuteronomy 32:43 AMP

Rejoice, O Gentiles, [with] His people; For He will avenge the blood of His servants, And render vengeance to His adversaries; He will provide atonement for His land [and] His people.
Deuteronomy 32:35 AMP

- God reserves vengeance for Himself. Why?

- Who might you hurt in your anger if you were to take vengeance yourself? (If you have taken vengeance in the past for your abortion pain, detail what happened).

Repentance for any sin must start at a personal level for it to spread. God is more than willing, ready and able to walk us through to forgiveness and reconciliation with Him, thereby repairing the damage that our abortion(s) caused. You might ask yourself, "What relationships do I have to repair?" Thinking it through, we can see that our relationship with God, ourselves, our sexual partners, our children, our parents and friends involved in the abortion were all affected. God sees what you have been through at the hands of others. He also sees the damage we ourselves have caused. Our abortion had a ripple effect on our entire life, but guess what? So will

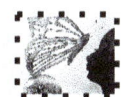

our healing! Remember, what the enemy meant for evil, God is working out for our good (Genesis 50:20).

Consider this verse from Acts 2:38 (AMP), *"And Peter said to them, 'Repent [change your old way of thinking, turn from your sinful ways, accept and follow Jesus as the Messiah] and be baptized, each of you, in the name of Jesus Christ for the forgiveness of your sins; and you will receive the gift of the Holy Spirit.'"*

- How would you know if you have received the gift of Holy Spirit?

- Who do you know Holy Spirit to be? (For assistance, see Isaiah 63:11; Matthew 1:18; Matthew 3:11; Mark 3:29; Mark 12:36; Mark 13:11).

- How has Holy Spirit shown up in your life?

- What Holy Spirit fruit would you like to bear as you shed the bitter fruits of anger, hate, bitterness, self-loathing, unforgiveness, guilt and shame?(see Galatians 5:22 to help you with identifying the fruit of the Spirit).

At this point in the study, you can see that the armor of "anger" we've used for so long was not effective or healthy. Instead, let us put on the armor of God as we move forward. His armor is a guaranteed multilayered level of protection that will only seek good and do no harm to the righteous. Ephesians 6:10-18 says that when the whole armor of God is fully deployed, we will be able to stand against the real enemy of our soul - the one that lied to us about our worth in God's eyes and about abortion.

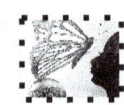

10 A final word: Be strong in the Lord and in his mighty power. 11 Put on all of God's armor so that you will be able to stand firm against all strategies of the devil. 12 For we are not fighting against flesh-and-blood enemies, but against evil rulers and authorities of the unseen world, against mighty powers in this dark world, and against evil spirits in the heavenly places. 13 Therefore, put on every piece of God's armor so you will be able to resist the enemy in the time of evil. Then after the battle you will still be standing firm. 14 Stand your ground, putting on the <u>belt of truth</u> and the <u>body armor of God's righteousness.</u> 15 For <u>shoes, put on the peace</u> that comes from the Good News so that you will be fully prepared. 16 In addition to all of these, hold up the <u>shield of faith</u> to stop the fiery arrows of the devil. 17 Put on <u>salvation as your helmet</u>, and take the <u>sword of the Spirit</u>, which is the word of God. 18 <u>Pray in the Spirit</u> at all times and on every occasion. Stay alert and be persistent in your prayers for all believers everywhere.

Ephesians 6:10-18

As we look at the pieces of armor God has given us, which piece(s) can you use this week to defeat the enemy attacks? Be as specific as you can with the help of Holy Spirit. It may help to personalize the verses from Ephesians by replacing "you" and "we" with "I".

Feel free to take a "praise break"

Let's continue Sis. Sylvia's story: I'd worn my mask for so long that I literally thought no one could see my spiritual pain. I was constantly acting out, seeking fleshly pleasures that weren't able to satisfy me. I was always so ANGRY for seemingly no reason; I didn't know enough to connect the dots to my abortion. My frequent nit-picking and outbursts at home eventually led to my separation from my husband. I thought every poor life-style choice I was making was because of an unhappy marriage. I was good at appearing calm,

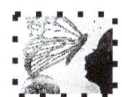

cool and collected in places where I had to be. But beneath the surface, where I hid my real feelings, it felt like an unbearable weight was pulling me down. My anger constantly bubbled up to the surface even after my separation; that was when I began to realize it wasn't nobody but me that I had to deal with. The numbness to my abortion was wearing off and the throbbing pain was setting in...

Let's tell our stories about our anger and the damage it caused. (talk about whatever came up for you in this chapter).

- How did telling your story make you feel?

- How could you relate to your sister's situation?

- What release have you felt from today's session?

Full Circle Moment of Reflection

Be still for a moment and reflect on what you have heard, read and experienced thus far. Be sure to journal about any stray emotions that continue to surface.

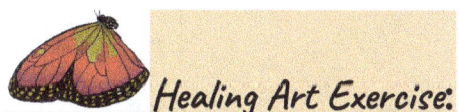

Healing Art Exercise: "The Iceberg"

Using an iceberg as a metaphor, we will explore our hidden emotions associated with anger. Click on the image for instructions in CANVA.

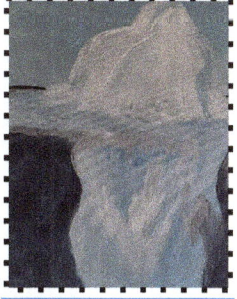

Sylvia Blakely 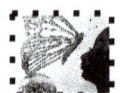 Arise, And Fly Free!

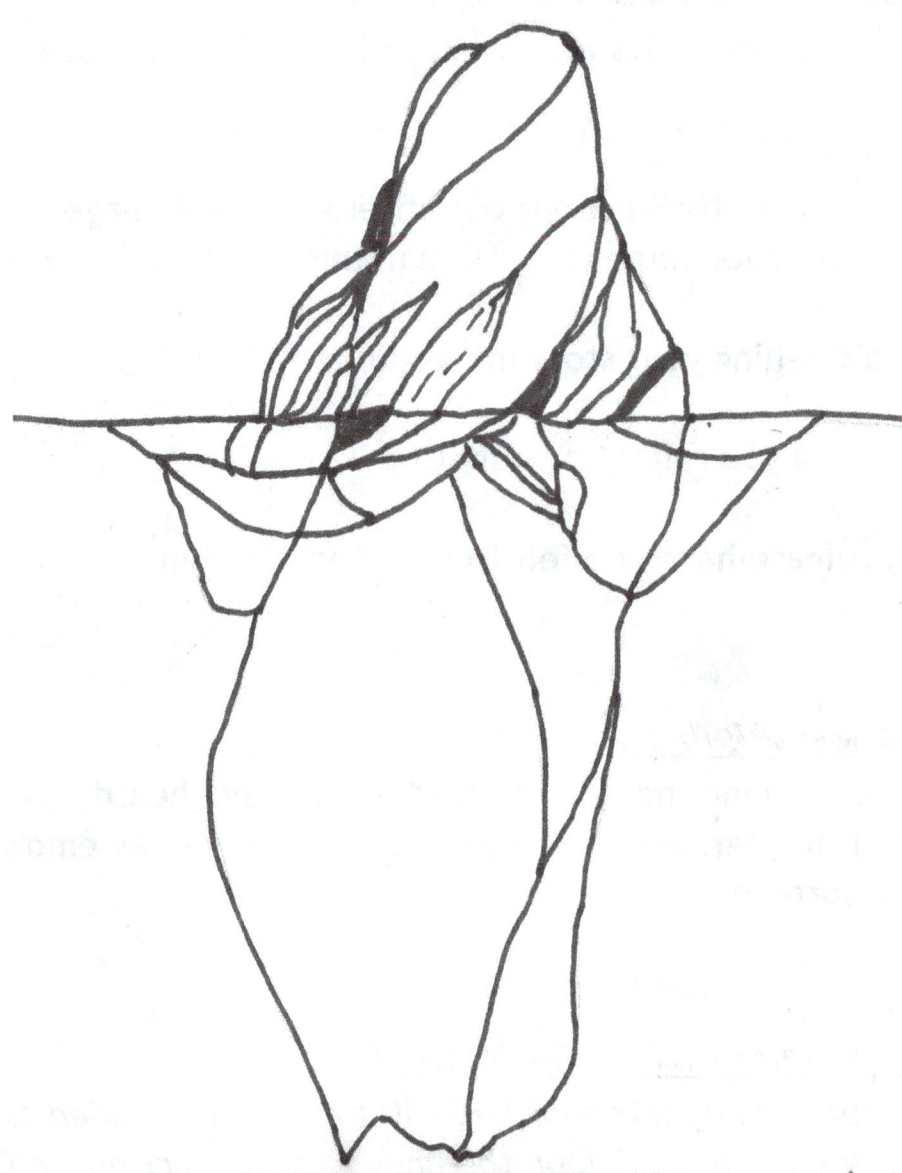

Printable Template by Roxy Fields

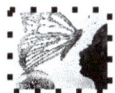

Write Your Prayer

Ask God to show you what being free of anger would look like and how to lay it at the foot of the cross. In addition, include a name of God or a characteristic of God that relates to you. Include three things you are grateful for.

Songs

- "Happy" by NF
- "He Kept Me" by Lamont Sanders.

Homework: WRITE Out YOUR Story

Include as much detail as you choose to. Write about what led up to your decision(s), the experience(s), how you felt afterwards, what God is doing to heal you and what you want others to know. Feel free to tape your story. Check in with your Wellness Team.

Notes:

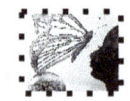

Chapter 6

Grieving Our Losses

"Would it be all right? Would it be all right to go ahead and feel? Go ahead and count on something?"
Beloved, 1998

In our country, we've been told repeatedly that abortion is no big deal and that there is no such thing as post-abortion sadness or regret. In fact, the most recent evil incarnation of this blasé attitude was a coffee mug I saw online that said, "Don't Even Talk to Me Until I've Had My Abortion." Once we look back a little ways, we can see the origin of a callousness about the life of the preborn and newborn that, although shocking now, was also seen as normal. In this country, not so very long ago, babies were openly bartered as a commodity. Neither mothers nor fathers had a say in where their offspring went after they were born. As Dr. Martin Luther King noted in his master work, Why We Can't Wait, "It is the emotionally remote American that has half forgotten the history of a system that bartered human beings."

Additionally, if an enslaved mother lost a child to miscarriage or stillbirth, she would not have had time to grieve for her child as her daily quota of work was still due. The enslavers' grief would have solely centered around the potential lost earnings that the child represented. The movie Beloved details a mother haunted by taking her own child's life. Rather than see her daughter placed in bondage she does the unthinkable and ends her life in what she considered a mercy killing. What happened then is still happening now in a way. When a modern mother sees her poverty akin to modern bondage, then we know this country still has a serious problem. We have not recognized, as a society, the need for the necessary resources to properly parent children. Billions of taxpayer dollars go towards limiting the birth of black children yet, only a fraction goes toward affordable housing, living wage jobs, low-cost child care etc. One mother stated, "I have to decide how I can afford another baby 'cause I know my other kids are gonna suffer. And that's not fair to them." In a country as affluent as America, the desire to have children should not be at financial odds with one's ability to parent.

We have a lot to grieve surrounding the inability to properly care for our children, both past and present.

As you allow yourself to think about and talk about your aborted child(ren), know that you have a right to grieve their loss, no matter the circumstances surrounding their death. It is entirely natural and spiritual for a woman to grieve the loss of her child(ren). Your child(ren) existed, no matter how briefly. They were assigned a sex at conception. They had a soul. You may have felt their presence. They might have even been given a name. Your child(ren) existed and they count no matter what past, present or future societal opinion exists about them. Opinions change but facts do not and, at the end of the day, your children are not here...but they mattered.

Watch: *Portraits of Grief in the Aftermath of Abortion* by Project Rachel.

BIBLE CONNECTION: Consider Bathsheba. As we read in 2 Samuel chapters 11 and 12, we see that sex outside of marriage between King David and Bathsheba was the sin which led to the birth of a child. We later learn that the Lord struck the child and he became sick and died. We never hear how Bathsheba dealt with all of this, especially the death of her son but in her place we can imagine unbearable pain. Bathsheba had a right to grieve the loss of her child because, at the end of the day, her child was gone; the circumstances of his birth and death did not matter.

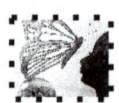

REFLECTION: OUR CHILDREN'S BRIEF LIVES COUNTED AND OUR GRIEF OVER THEIR LOSS HAS MEANING WHETHER OR NOT THAT GRIEF WAS ACKNOWLEDGED. GRIEF, EVEN WHEN IT IS NOT ACKNOWLEDGED BY SOCIETY, IS STILL VALID.

 *What Does God Have to Say?*

This is what the LORD says: "A cry is heard in Ramah--deep anguish and bitter weeping. Rachel weeps for her children, refusing to be comforted-- for her children are gone."
Jeremiah 31:15

For many of us, there was a state of relief that overcame us after the abortion(s). It is hard to write that but it is nonetheless true. No loud weeping or wailing occurred after our abortion(s) because there was a denial of the humanity of our child(ren). There may have been a sense of relief after the abortion(s) because it seemed that a temporary problem was resolved or future catastrophe was avoided. There may have been relief because, at the time, resources were scarce and support from family and friends was minimal. Relief may have come because you felt you were honoring the wishes of the father of the baby to abort. In your mind at the time, you may have felt that a relationship with the baby would block a future relationship with the father or that you could not raise your child without him supporting you.

There is no condemnation for the "why" of your choice.

But, now that abortion regret has surfaced and replaced the sense of relief, we are forced to acknowledge the trauma that was done to our soul. This type of grief weighs heavy on the heart. The emotions that could no longer be suppressed have bobbed up to the surface and have now demanded our attention.

Often, the emotions we feel are not recognized as grief initially. For many of us, we sensed anger first because we could not find a readily identifiable cause. Once the numbness wore off, volcanoes of anger erupted all over us (and the people closest to us) leaving melted relationships in its wake. What we want to be able to do is cry for our lost child(ren). Like Rachel, our soul refuses to be comforted until it is allowed to grieve. There may be a part of you that feels you do not have a right to grieve; my sister, that is a lie from the enemy of your soul! Know that the enemy's whole objective is to steal, kill and destroy (John 10:10) the existence and memory of your child(ren). The comfort you deserve will only come at the hands of the lover of your soul, Jesus Christ Himself.

God, our gracious heavenly Father, is giving you permission to grieve. Cry for your child(ren) not here. Cry for lost relationships be they with the father or with family. Cry because you didn't trust your intuition. Cry because you didn't change your mind. Cry because you did, yet you still went through with it. Cry because you didn't run out of the clinic. Cry because you believed the lies you were told. Cry because you didn't look at the ultrasound. Cry because you saw your child and you still went through with it. Cry because you didn't trust God to see you through and now, you wished you had.

It is OK to cry...Stop and take a break if needed... Let this song by Koryn Hawthorne minister to you. "Cry."

- How has it felt to finally be able to acknowledge and cry for your child(ren)?

- If you could write a lament or a sad song for your child(ren) what words would you include? (Use the books of Psalms and Lamentations for inspiration.)

- For many of us, grief has been a very private affair. To learn more about quiet grief, we recommend the book,

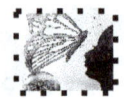

"Encouragement for Those Who Suffer in Silence" by Rev. Dr. LaRuth E. Lockhart.

"Then I will pour out a spirit of grace and prayer on the family of David and on the people of Jerusalem. They will look on me whom they have pierced and mourn for him as for an only son. They will grieve bitterly for him as for a firstborn son who has died.
Zechariah 12:10

- Your aborted child may have been your first born, an only son or daughter, twins etc. How does this acknowledgement affect your grief?

- How does the title of *mother* to your aborted child(ren) sit with you? Explain in detail.

- If you have never given birth after your abortion(s), how has that affected you? Describe in detail.

In the book of Ruth Chapter 4, Verses 13-17, Ruth's mother-in-law Naomi is honored by her friends because of the birth of Ruth's son, Obed. Grandparents, siblings, aunts and uncles are significant family roles that are affected by abortion(s); ones which we may not always acknowledge.

- Who else in your circle has missed out on the grief process associated with the loss of your child? Name them and their relationship to your child(ren).

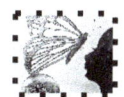

- Have you talked with those in your circle who also experienced the loss of your child(ren)? If no, why not?

- Can you feel the spirit of grace that God has poured out on you in your grief? If yes, how? If not, why?

Let's take a moment to read and reflect on the story of King David in 2 Samuel 11:1-27 and look for parallels to our stories.

- What part did lust play in the story?

- How did sex outside of marriage set the stage?

- Why did the king find it necessary - in his mind - to commit murder?

In 2 Samuel 12:1-23, King David's story continues to unfold. Read the passages and reflect on the following questions:

- What series of events did it take to get David's attention about what he'd done?

- How do you interpret the death of the child?

- What action did David take that showed his remorse?

- Has your relationship with the father of your baby survived the abortion? How has the relationship status affected your grief?

- It is said that grief can spiral into despair. Look up the definition of both *grief* and *despair*. What is the difference in meaning?

- What did King David say about his child after his death that was hopeful?

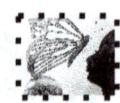

- Do you believe you will see your child(ren) again? Why or why not?

To all who mourn in Israel, he will give a crown of beauty for ashes, a joyous blessing instead of mourning, festive praise instead of despair. In their righteousness, they will be like great oaks that the LORD has planted for his own glory.
Isaiah 61:3

Beloved, God has a different outcome planned for you than the one you may think you deserve. It might not feel like it now but, there is a new force on the horizon; one almost as powerful as love and that is *hope*. Once you take hold of the promises in Isaiah 61:3 a whole new world will appear. There is a purpose for the grief we feel and there is a rejoicing that will come out of it that is hard to imagine right now. Just hold on! God is not through with you yet! Know how I know? Because God has not gotten the glory yet for your healing!

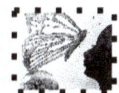

Check In: "The Wail"

Prepare a soft place to sit, get a pillow and for 10 or so seconds, cry out, as loud as you can, into the pillow (you might want to warn others within ear shot beforehand). Repeat until you are worn out. Then, relax and cry out as you are led to.

Expert Opinion: Grief
- Article: "What's Your Grief?" by Litsa Williams
- Biblical Grief: The Book of Lamentations by the Bible Project

Let's hear more of Sis. Sylvia's story: God brought a woman into my life who showed me His unconditional love. She was a mother of two, a wife, a devoted church goer and an example of the best of Christianity. I returned to church and joined a small group who showed me how to follow Christ in a way that would please Him. I began to volunteer at a Pregnancy Resource Center once my husband and I moved to a small town in Ohio. I loved teaching abstinence to middle and high school kids hoping to avert sexual activity before marriage or at least renew a commitment to abstinence. But, I noticed it was still hard for me to talk about abortion and I knew I couldn't work in the clinic with the ultrasound machine because it was just "too much." I started melting down every Mother's Day and I was always so angry but I didn't understand why. The pain of my abortion was not healed and so I suffered everytime I bumped up against a trigger such as a newborn baby. I even suffered my way through dental appointments not realizing that the position of the chair and the oral suction were triggers. I was beginning the grief process but I didn't know that at the time. This went on for another 20 years.

Let's take time to tell our story of when we first felt the loss of our child(ren).

- How did telling your story make you feel?

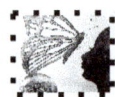

- How could you relate to your sister's difficulty in grieving?

- Have feelings of depression or suicidal thoughts come up for you? If so, who have you spoken to regarding your feelings?

Here are three resources if you are experiencing depression or suicidal thoughts:
   - H3Helpline.org for 24/7 peer support.
   - 988 Suicide & Crisis Lifeline. Call or text 24/7 for counseling.
   - Focus on the Family Hotline: 800-232-6459, for free or low cost counseling.

Full Circle Moment of Reflection

Be still for a moment and reflect on what you have heard, read and experienced thus far. Feel free to share your homework, *Letter to Your Bestie*. Use your journal as a means of reflection.

Healing Art Exercise: "Who and What is Missing?"

Find a family photo you like. Sit with it and envision where an additional person(s) would be. Who might they look like and where might they be placed in the family photo? Journal any thoughts or feelings that come to the surface.

Sylvia Blakely 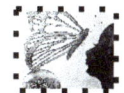 Arise, And Fly Free!

Write Your Prayer

Ask God to share with you the sex and name of your child(ren). Ask earnestly, be patient and listen intently. Include one of the names of God or a characteristic of God in your prayer. Include three things you are grateful for.

Song

- *"Made in the Image of God"* by We Are Messengers.

Homework:

Continue to work on writing a lament OR choose a lament from the book of Lamentations or Psalms that expresses your feelings.

Notes:

Chapter 7

Forgiving the Unforgivable

"It's one of the greatest gifts you can give yourself: to forgive. Forgive everybody." Maya Angelou

There are so many difficult aspects of our abortion that we may see as unforgivable. Between societal and other factors, we see now that we were sold a web of lies about abortion. According to society, no one dies in an abortion so, what is the big deal? But now that abortion guilt and shame have finally come to the surface, we may sometimes feel underwater with God. "How can God forgive the 'unforgivable' sin of abortion? Aren't You all about justice, God? And if You are then, don't I deserve death?"

We can sometimes make the mistake of taking on the job of weighing out sins. It's as if we say to God, "I know exactly how each of our sins grieve You and what the punishment should be." It is true that God did not intend for abortion to happen but, make no mistake: all sin grieves God's heart! A good question to ask at this juncture might be, "why would God need a mechanism (forgiveness) to make things right if He hadn't anticipated that things would go wrong?" Remember the characteristics of God that say He is faithful and just? Romans 6:23 NLT]23 *For the wages of sin is death, but the free gift of God is eternal life through Christ Jesus our Lord.*

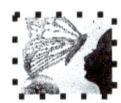

God's mechanism for forgiving any sin starts with His children acknowledging AND confessing their sin. 1 John 1:9 AMP says *9 If we [freely] admit that we have sinned and confess our sins, He is faithful and just [true to His own nature and promises], and will forgive our sins and cleanse us continually from all unrighteousness [our wrongdoing, everything not in conformity with His will and purpose].*

God and only God can do the work of forgiveness because He is the only one who can use His grace and mercy to literally blot out our sins and cleanse us. We do not have the capacity to weigh out sin or to weigh out forgiveness; those jobs belong to God and God alone.

Jesus taught His disciples a prayer that would continually remind them that forgiveness was a gift granted by God when requested, but that forgiveness involved us doing for others what God was gracious enough to do to us. Matthew 6:12 AMP, *12 'And forgive us our debts, as we have forgiven our debtors [letting go of both the wrong and the resentment].* As we explored in chapter five, all of the negative emotions that we hold onto (which include those towards ourselves) cannot be healed if they are not released in confession to God. The Lord is listening out for our hearts to cry! We may know that our behaviors leading up to the abortion were sins as well but we have not yet confessed those. My sister, it is time to come clean and with deep humility confess it all; the fornication, the lies, the manipulation, the hiding, the cooperation in the abortion act, all of it. Verse 10 of first John 1:1 says, *10 If we say that we have not sinned [refusing to admit acts of sin], we make Him [out to be] a liar [by contradicting Him] and His word is not in us.*

Believe it or not, God was looking out for both you and your child(ren) prior to the abortion. We may have missed the ways He provided for our escape but, He does not want you to miss out on His offer of forgiveness. The only thing standing in the way of your release from the muck and mire is your rejection of His gift of forgiveness. You may not feel worthy of the gift or the gift may actually make you feel worse which would be totally understandable given what we have done. But, it may ease your mind to know that you really don't deserve the gift; none of us do. I didn't. It is simply in God's Holy nature to present it to us anyway because He loves us (Read Psalms 130:3-5 for spiritual support). God was prepared for our sin, not pleased by it. God would much rather a sinner repent than to die and so He gives us chances! Ezekial 33:11 NLT 11 *As surely as I live, says the Sovereign LORD, I take no pleasure in the death of wicked people. I only want them to turn from their wicked ways so they can live. Turn! Turn from your wickedness, O people of Israel! Why should you die?*

God loves us so much that He sent His only Son to die on behalf of the sins we would commit including abortion. As Christ followers we can accept the fact that we did not deserve what He did on the cross for us. We have to trust however, that the blood He shed on the cross was sufficient to cover our sin of abortion(s) OR His blood didn't cover any sin. Period. Stay here a minute until that last sentence sinks deep into your heart…

BIBLE CONNECTION: THE STORY OF SAPPHIRA IN THE BOOK OF ACTS IS MEMORABLE FOR THE SWIFT JUSTICE GOD CAN BRING ON UNREPENTANT SINNERS (ACTS 4:32-5:11). HERE WAS A WOMAN WHO CHOSE TO CONSPIRE WITH HER HUSBAND ANANIAS AND LIE TO GOD. AS WE LOOK AT THE STORY, HUSBAND AND WIFE WERE CALLED IN SEPARATELY TO SEE THE APOSTLES ABOUT THE PROCEEDS ON THE SALE OF A PIECE OF PROPERTY THEY OWNED. EACH OF THEM WERE GIVEN A CHANCE TO TELL HOW THEY SOLD THE LAND AND CONFESS TO WHAT HAPPENED TO THE MONEY PROMISED TO THE CHURCH. SAPPHIRA STUCK WITH THE CONSPIRACY TO GO BACK ON A VOW AND SHE REFUSED THE ESCAPE ROUTE AND THE CHANCE FOR REPENTANCE AND FORGIVENESS THAT WAS OFFERED TO HER. THE STORY CONCLUDES THAT SHE PAID FOR HER CHOICE WITH HER LIFE AS DID HER HUSBAND BEFORE HER. REFLECTION: GOD GIVES US OPPORTUNITIES TO REPENT AFTER WE MAKE A GRAVE ERROR. HOW OFTEN DO WE DIG OUR OWN SPIRITUAL GRAVE BY IGNORING HIM?

Let's look at the story of Joseph in Genesis beginning in chapter 37. Joseph was sold into slavery but eventually became second in command in Egypt. Joseph had every reason to not extend grace and mercy to his family after the way he was treated by his brothers. But God allowed him to see that what he endured would come together for good and so, Joseph chose to forgive. Through that act of forgiveness, a covenant promise was fulfilled and a nation was spared.

'Thus you shall say to Joseph: "I beg you, please forgive the trespass of your brothers and their sin; for they did evil to you." ' Now, please, forgive the trespass of the servants of the God of your father." And Joseph wept when they spoke to him.
Genesis 50:17 NKJV

- Why is it important to actually ask for forgiveness from everyone done wrong by the abortion(s)?

- Why is it important to have someone else bear witness to your actions of forgiveness?

Then if my people who are called by my name will humble themselves and pray and seek my face and turn from their wicked ways, I will hear from heaven and will forgive their sins and restore their land.
2 Chronicles 7:14

- Why is humility important to God?

- What other aspects of this verse speak to you?

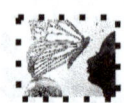

35 "If the skies are shut up and there is no rain because your people have sinned against you, and if they pray toward this Temple and acknowledge your name and turn from their sins because you have punished them, 36 then hear from heaven and forgive the sins of your servants, your people Israel. Teach them to follow the right path, and send rain on your land that you have given to your people as their special possession.

1 Kings 8: 35-36

- Up till now, you may have been feeling stuck, unable to move forward because of your unconfessed sin. What is the way forward as you understand the verses from 1 Kings?

- What *healing rain* can you envision God might be holding for you?

Feel my pain and see my trouble. Forgive all my sins.
Psalm 25:18

- How has God shown you that He sees your pain?

- Asking for forgiveness from God and feeling that you have been forgiven by God can be drastically different things. How do you think you will know that God has answered your request for forgiveness?

Because of your anger, my whole body is sick; my health is broken because of my sins.
Psalm 38:3

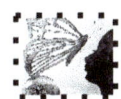

- How important is it to be seen and heard on this healing journey? By God? By others?

- Do you believe that God has seen your pain all along? If yes, what was the evidence?

- When we ask for forgiveness of our sins, how do we know that includes our abortion(s)?

And they will not need to teach their neighbors, nor will they need to teach their relatives, saying, 'You should know the Lord.' For everyone, from the least to the greatest, will know me already," says the Lord. "And I will forgive their wickedness, and I will never again remember their sins."
Jeremiah 31:34

- It's been said that each of us has a *God-sized* hole in our hearts. How does this verse support that AND give us hope?

- Does God acknowledge us even when we don't acknowledge Him? Why or why not?

- God says that not only will He forgive our sin, but that He will not remember it. How can you trust that passage?

12 and forgive us our sins, as we have forgiven those who sin against us. 13 And don't let us yield to temptation, but rescue us from the evil one. 14 "If you forgive those who sin against you, your heavenly Father will forgive you. 15 But if you refuse to forgive others, your Father will not forgive your sins.
Matthew 6:12, 14-15

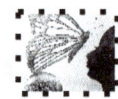

- Who on your list of offenders is forgiven? Who is not? Why?

- Why do you think Jesus included *forgiveness* in the prayer He taught His disciples?

- Is forgiveness conditional? Why or why not?

- Why does Jesus command us not to judge or to condemn?

- True forgiveness comes from a changed heart. Explain.

3 So watch yourselves! "If another believer sins, rebuke that person; then if there is repentance, forgive. 4 Even if that person wrongs you seven times a day and each time turns again and asks forgiveness, you must forgive."
Luke 17:3-4

- Some may interpret Luke 17:3-4 as an opportunity for someone to abuse you or take advantage of you. Why is that not the case?

- Repentance has to happen for forgiveness to be genuine. Explain.

- How does that relate to where you are in your story of forgiving yourself for the abortion(s)?

But if we confess our sins to him, he is faithful and just to forgive us our sins and to cleanse us from all wickedness.
1 John 1:9

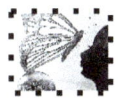

- Whose faithfulness is our forgiveness dependent upon?

10 When you forgive this man, I forgive him, too. And when I forgive whatever needs to be forgiven, I do so with Christ's authority for your benefit, 11 so that Satan will not outsmart us. For we are familiar with his evil schemes.
2 Corinthians 2:10-11

- Why does Paul urge fellow Christ followers to forgive one another even if they themselves were not directly offended?

- Does the person you forgive have to accept the gift of forgiveness?

"I--yes, I alone--will blot out your sins for my own sake and will never think of them again.
Isaiah 43:25

- As our sins are erased, how does that pave the way for a different type of relationship with God?

Take a look at the video: *"God's Consistent Posture"* by BibleProject. (about 5 minutes).

- What is it about the character of God that would remove and forget sins?

Therefore if anyone is in Christ [that is, grafted in, joined to Him by faith in Him as Savior], he is a new creature [reborn and renewed by the Holy Spirit]; the old things [the previous moral and spiritual condition] have passed away. Behold, new things have come [because spiritual awakening brings a new life].
2 Corinthians 5:17 AMP

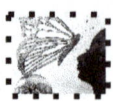

- How do we receive the gift of renewal God offers us?

- If God can and has forgiven you, have you extended the gift of forgiveness to yourself? Why or why not?

- Going back to the statement by Maya Angelou at the beginning of the chapter: *"It's one of the greatest gifts you can give yourself: to forgive. Forgive everybody."* answer this last question: Who is capable of offering forgiveness, who is forgiveness really for and why?

Check In: "Full Body Relaxation". Let the emotions flow...Continue to access our Wellness Basket.

Expert Opinion
- Watch "Soul Care For Today's Woman" by Dr. Barbara Peacock and why it is important (34 minutes).
- "Forgiveness" by Voddie Baucham (50 minutes)
- "Forgive and Extend An Act Of Kindness" on Better Together with Priscilla Shirer 10 minutes.
- Watch Tyler Perry talk about the power of forgiveness. 3 minutes.

Let's continue with Sylvia's story: Once I'd experienced God's unconditional love through my co-worker, I decided to return to church and regular worship services. I was literally loved back to life and into a deep relationship with God to where I was FINALLY able to ask for His forgiveness for my abortion. Of course, God said, "yes daughter, you are forgiven" and I felt His love wash over me immediately! God began to move in my heart in a totally new way and so much of my anger and stony heart began to be replaced by flesh. I felt forgiven by God but, it took going through healing for me to admit that I had not accepted the gift of forgiveness for myself. I recognized that although the Lord had released me from my jail cell, I hadn't walked out into the fresh air...

- Could you relate to this part of Sylvia's story?

- How has unforgiveness kept you bound?

Full Circle Moment of Reflection

What does it mean to truly extend the gift of forgiveness to yourself and others? Be still for a moment and reflect on what you have heard, read and experienced thus far. Be sure to journal about any stray emotions (like anger) that continue to surface.

Art Exercise: "Mirror Affirmations."

Using a mirror, take 15 minutes to really look at yourself without judgment. Write down key words that God is speaking to you through Holy Spirit. Make "I am" statements of faith. For example you might write, "I am worthy of forgiveness."

Write Out Your Prayer

Ask God to help you with any residual unforgiveness in your heart towards anyone (including yourself or God). Include one of the names of God or a characteristic of God in your prayer. Include three things you are grateful for.

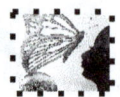

Songs
- "Beautiful Savior" by Tasha Page-Lockhart (feat. Bryan Popin).
- "Great Work" by Brian Courtney Wilson.

Homework: Work on the Memorial for your child(ren).

Complete the baby information card if you are able. Our group memorial will focus on the theme, "Setting a Place At the Table." Begin to gather together items to mark a place at the dinner table for your child(ren). Check in with your Wellness Team and share your progress.

Chapter 8

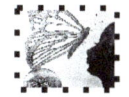

Restoring Hope

"Well son, I'll tell you: Life for me ain't been no crystal stair. It's had tacks in it, And splinters, And boards torn up, And places with no carpet on the floor- Bare. But all the time I'se been a-climbin' on, And reachin' landin's, And turnin' corners, And sometimes goin' in the dark Where there ain't been no light. So boy, don't you turn back. Don't you set down on the steps "Cause you finds it's kinder hard. Don't you fall now- For I'se still goin', honey, I'se still climbin', And life for me ain't been no crystal stair."
"Mother to Son" by Langston Hughes

"Mother to Son", one of Langston Hughes' most well known works, stands as a tribute to the strength of those who kept climbing despite the odds. This poem drips with hope and possibility despite hardships. Hope is one of the most powerful forces a woman can employ. Hope kept a people starved of food and knowledge alive. Hope beat back the despair that crept up in the middle of the night as enslavers did whatever they wanted to the enslaved. The act of hope is the purest act of faith in that there is a belief that current circumstances can and will change in the future. It can be said that when man loses hope, he loses his humanity. Lesser animals may trust in instinct, but man employs hope as an even more powerful tool. This generation of free individuals stands on the hopes of men and women brought here in chains; that is something deep to ponder and something real to hold onto.

There is hope rising in our country surrounding the sanctity and sacredness of life from the "womb to the tomb." Many Christian young women and men are rejecting the worn out mantras of "Our Body, Our Choice." Young people are beginning to understand that they in fact have been physically and spiritually bought with a price that is beyond valuation. First Corinthians 6:20 says, *"for God bought you with a high price. So you must honor God with your body."*

Our opportunity to glorify God is restorable as we reconcile ourselves to God. Remember King David's horrible misstep with Bathsheba and the resultant death of his son? (2 Samuel 12:8-23). Once David heard about and then acknowledged his son's death, he did something his courtiers didn't expect: he washed up, worshiped God and broke his fast. He then went to be with the person with whom he had committed the sin (Bathsheba) and God blessed them with another son named Solomon.

God is in the business of restoring relationships. Once He calls you His child, He will move whatever needs to be moved - including the stone in your own heart - to commune with you (Read Ezekiel 36:26-27 for spiritual inspiration). After all, He made the ultimate sacrifice of His Son while we were yet still sinning (Romans 5:8). If we accept this gift of God's grace and mercy, it will purely be an act of faith on our part. If God is who He says He is, and He can do what He says He can do, then we are forgiven if we are willing to accept what He is offering us. Make no mistake, there is nothing this book can do to save you. It can only point you to the One who can. Repentance from our sins and acceptance of God's saving mercy and grace are commitments made in the heart and walked out in faith. You simply have to hope and put in the work knowing that your future will be better and brighter than your past.

Let that settle in... Seriously. Pray into it. Journal about it. Share with a godly sister or brother and know that you know that you know that God has given you the gift of His forgiveness. And with that, you can finally, FINALLY accept His gift and forgive yourself.

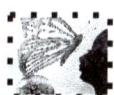

BIBLE CONNECTION: Consider the redemption of Mary Magdalene by Jesus in Luke 8:1-2. Mary was healed and cleansed of serious demonic possession. Jesus cast out not one but seven demons from a woman who would become a devoted disciple and supporter. What must Mary have endured when she was possessed by a legion? We can't know for sure but certainly at this point we may be able to relate to living with the enemies' lies for far too long as Mary did. The bible does not say that Mary dwelt on her past and we never hear another disciple attach her past to her present. On the contrary, she was trusted as a true disciple and was one of first to hear the good news of Christ's resurrection in Mark 16:9. As far as we know, Mary's hope was restored and she served Jesus without reservation or restriction. Mary was given one of the most powerful forces in our human world and that is hope!

REFLECTION: Once God restores hope that you can be healed from the pain of your abortion you can serve him without reservation as Mary did.

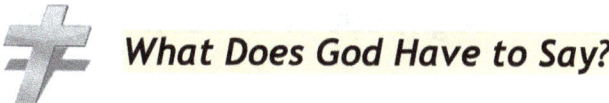

What Does God Have to Say?

Who Does God Say You Are?

- "You Are Who God Says You Are" by Priscilla Shirer. 13 minutes.

When God brought Abram out of the land of Ur, Abram decided to put his hope and trust in the God who spoke to him. He had to have faith that what God said would happen would come to pass. When God made covenants with Abram and blessed him repeatedly, Abram could only hope and trust that, even though he wouldn't be alive to witness all that God promised, it would still happen. Abraham was credited with having faith built upon hope and trust in a future he could not see because He trusted The One who held the future. Make no mistake, Abraham made some questionable decisions along the way. God restored hope each and every time by renewing their relationship and reminding him of the plan.

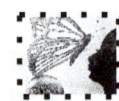

Never doubt that you will be healed from the pain of your abortion. Like Abraham, you may go through a few ups and downs and make plenty of mistakes to get to where God promised He would take you; but know that you will arrive. As our gracious Lord restores His relationship with us, we have renewed hope. With hope, there is a sense of peace that everything will work together for good. Your wounds may heal with a visible scar but that will be someone's invitation to ask about your story.

You intended to harm me, but God intended it all for good. He brought me to this position so I could save the lives of many people.
Genesis 50:20

- What good has been brought out of the evil of your abortion(s)?

- How does that *good* give God glory?

Surely your goodness and unfailing love will pursue me all the days of my life, and I will live in the house of the LORD forever.
Psalm 23:6

- Can you recall a time when either *goodness and mercy* followed you?

- What statement of faith is David making?

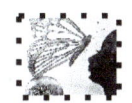

25 The LORD says, "I will give you back what you lost to the swarming locusts, the hopping locusts, the stripping locusts, and the cutting locusts. It was I who sent this great destroying army against you. 26 Once again you will have all the food you want, and you will praise the LORD your God, who does these miracles for you. Never again will my people be disgraced. 27 Then you will know that I am among my people Israel, that I am the LORD your God, and there is no other. Never again will my people be disgraced.
Joel 2:25-27 says

God is a God of restoration! No matter the how, why, when or where of your loss, God is in the business of bringing us back into a love relationship with Him. He does this because it gives Him pleasure to do so.

- What part of your identity was put to shame because of your abortion(s)?

- What areas of your life do you want the Lord to restore? For example, do you feel like a mother to your aborted child(ren).

Isaiah 38: 17 AMP "Indeed, it was for my own well-being that I had such bitterness; But You have loved back my life from the pit of nothingness (destruction), For You have cast all my sins behind Your back.

- What might the restoration process look like going forward?

Sylvia Blakely

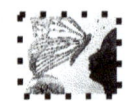

Arise, And Fly Free!

Check In: Box Breathing

Expert Opinion

Let's finish hearing Sis. Sylvia's story: I was later introduced to abortion healing (which I didn't even know existed!) once we moved to Florida. I took a healing course that finally set me free in a way that allowed me to honor God by starting the Arise Daughter and Arise Artists ministries. I was given the gift of knowing the sex and name of my baby (Ellen Francis) and the confidence that she is now being cared for by Jesus and that I will see her again.

These next two verses from the prophet Isaiah nourished me and kept me under the shadow of The Fathers wings: Isaiah 60:1 New King James Version:

"Arise, shine; For your light has come! And the glory of the LORD is risen upon you."
Isaiah 60:1 NKJV.

"The Spirit of the Lord GOD [is] upon Me, Because the LORD has anointed Me To preach good tidings to the poor; He has sent Me to heal the brokenhearted, To proclaim liberty to the captives, And the opening of the prison to [those who are] bound; 2 To proclaim the acceptable year of the LORD, And the day of vengeance of our God; To comfort all who mourn, 3 To console those who mourn in Zion, To give them beauty for ashes, The oil of joy for mourning, The garment of praise for the spirit of heaviness; That they may be called trees of righteousness, The planting of the LORD, that He may be glorified."
Isaiah 61: 1-3 NKJV

I was renewed, restored, reconciled and given a mandate to carry forth the ministry of reconciliation (2 Corinthians 5:17-19) and to comfort those as I had been comforted ([2 Corinthians 1:4](#)). God used it all for good ([Romans 8:28](#)) and for those great gifts of forgiveness and freedom I will be forever grateful.

Let's hear YOUR WRITTEN story about how God is restoring you. Start with your name, your age at the time of the abortion and your age now, and how the Lord brought you to this place of healing. What do you want others to know? Include an acknowledgement to your child(ren).

- How did your sister's story make you feel?

- What aspects of her story could you relate to?

- What has been the hardest part about forgiving yourself?

Full Circle Moment of Reflection

Be still for a moment and reflect on what you have heard, read and experienced thus far. Take time to write in your journal what has been revealed to you. *We will take a 15 minute break prior to the memorial service. Feel free to go off camera to prepare*

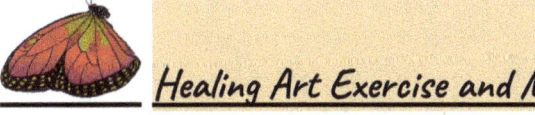 *Healing Art Exercise and Memorial:* "Let's Set the Family Table" * A special thank you to Ms. Schearice Moore for this idea.

Let's take some time to bring our child(ren) back into the family. Let's set a table with a place for them as an acknowledgment of their continued presence in our hearts. Let's take a picture of our now complete family dinner table as a sweet reminder of how God restores.

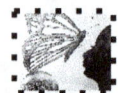

Write Your Prayer

Thank God for the *good* that you have received through your healing journey. Include one of the names of God or a characteristic of God. Include three things you are grateful for.

Songs

- "Worth Fighting For" by Brian Courtney Wilson.
- "For My Good" by Todd Galberth.
- "Sea of Forgetfulness" by Helen Baylor.

Homework:

Go to: optionline.org and locate the nearest Pregnancy Resource Center.

Notes:

Chapter 9

Walking In Freedom!

"I thank God for my journey
And I wouldn't go back.
There's a rhythm to the struggle
There's no 'half' and no 'slack'.
You're full in or full out
It takes discipline, no lack.
I thank God for my journey
And I'm not going back."

"My Journey" by Sylvia Blakely

God intended for us to live in a covenant state of holy matrimony with a man whom we love and can enjoy a rich sex life with. A life lived outside of God's intentions is a life filled with avoidable consequences (as we have already discussed in detail). When we have sex outside of the marriage covenant, we are essentially creating bonds with multiple "false husbands." As you recall the story of Jesus and the Samaritan woman at the well in the Gospel of John, chapter 4, verses 1-43, note that Jesus acknowledged the woman's past and current situation without condemning her. No doubt, she was already aware of the religious laws that should have governed her behavior. By Jesus going out of His way to lovingly confront the woman at the well about her "false husbands", He was able to both convict her behavior and ignite her faith in Him in the same encounter; what a mighty and gracious God we serve!

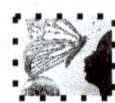

Jesus knows our past sexual sins and He has come near to you to both convict and forgive. When we accept His gift we walk out our freedom. And with freedom comes responsibility which God wants us to use wisely.

Bible connection: The story of the unnamed woman caught in the act of adultery (John 8:1-11) is an often told cautionary tale. Jesus came to the temple that day to teach and teach He did! He taught man to not judge hastily especially if you yourself have not repented of your own sins. He taught what grace and mercy in action looked like. He taught that sins should not be repeated once repented of. He taught that his love was the law in action.

Reflection: Once God has shut your abusers and accusers down, you can live in freedom from the bondage of sin. Recognize that his grace came at a great cost and that freedom has great responsibilities. My sister, go and sin no more!

 **What Does God Have to Say?**

3 As he was speaking, the teachers of religious law and the Pharisees brought a woman who had been caught in the act of adultery. They put her in front of the crowd. 4 "Teacher," they said to Jesus, "this woman was caught in the act of adultery.
John 8: 3-4

When Jesus was confronted at the temple with a woman accused by the scribes and Pharisees of adultery in the Gospel of John, Chapter 8, Verses 1-11, Jesus was simultaneously accusing the sinful men who brought her before Him. Make no mistake, Jesus did not miss any of the subtleties of this situation. In these verses, we witness Christ's compassion and protection for the woman. Jesus also makes it crystal clear that she was only half of the adulterous equation

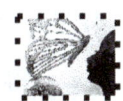

because she couldn't have committed adultery alone. However, as we recall the story (secretly enjoying Jesus' *clap back*), we often stop short of reciting the '*b*' part of verse 11 where Christ issues an admonishment to the woman to "Go and sin no more." Christ knows it takes two to commit adultery, but He is clearly trusting the woman, whose life is literally on the line, to repent (turn from), and change her behavior. Yes, sketchy sexual situations will continue to arise in our lives but Jesus is giving us the power to do things differently. The men in our lives may not choose to change their behavior but that doesn't mean we have to fall for their shenanigans. Remember: your power has been given back to you by the Redeemer of the universe! Reclaim your worth daughter of the Most High God for you have an amazing future planned for you; one where you can experience true love and security as God originally planned it out.

4 "Haven't you read the Scriptures?" Jesus replied. "They record that from the beginning 'God made them male and female.' 5 And he said, 'This explains why a man leaves his father and mother and is joined to his wife, and the two are united into one.' 6 Since they are no longer two but one, let no one split apart what God has joined together."
Matthew 19:4-6

- As we look deeper into how God wants us to proceed from here, lets consider the significance of a man leaving his family and joining with yours? How is this move meant to be of value for women?

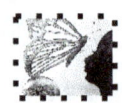

16 And don't you realize that if a man joins himself to a prostitute, he becomes one body with her? For the Scriptures say, "The two are united into one."... 18 Run from sexual sin! No other sin so clearly affects the body as this one does. For sexual immorality is a sin against your own body.
1 Corinthians 6:16,18

- It has been said that when we have sex with someone, we are actually having sex with everyone else they have ever had sex with. How does that make you feel?

- Men are hardwired to be protective of the woman they physically and emotionally bond with. How is God's design beneficial towards us as women?

- What are the benefits for men to refrain from sex until marriage?

31 Jesus said to the people who believed in him, "You are truly my disciples if you remain faithful to my teachings. 32 And you will know the truth, and the truth will set you free."... 34 Jesus replied, "I tell you the truth, everyone who sins is a slave of sin. A slave is not a permanent member of the family, but a son is part of the family forever. 36 So if the Son sets you free, you are truly free.
John 8:31-32, 34-36

Jesus has the same intentions for us as His Father does. God did not send His Son to condemn us (John 3:17). Jesus did not condemn the women He encountered in the courtyard or the one by the well. But, He is calling us back to righteousness through repentance and salvation. God wants that free and intimate Eden experience with us here on earth and into eternity through His Son Jesus Christ. We have

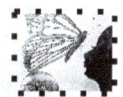

to be willing to live right (God's way) so that we are no longer ruled by the culture (sinful nature) of man but by the Kingdom of God.

    Rebelliousness to God's way of doing things can be very stealthy. As much as we hate to admit it, each of us is vulnerable to the pull of eroding cultural norms. Just take a look at some of our old sitcoms for example. It is easy to see what looked normal back then in comparison to now in terms of sexual mores. How far have we drifted in our own lifetime? With spiritual eyes open, we can begin to see how the enemy of our soul has attempted to steal, kill and destroy our hopes and dreams little by little. When we operate outside of God's plan we invite chaos. When we listen to man and ignore God, our lives become unnecessarily messy.   Thank God, His plan for redemption is perfect!

- How are we responsible for following Jesus's teaching as it concerns our bodies?

- What shackles are you willing to remove from your mind in regards to who you should follow - man or God? Be specific.

We know that our old sinful selves were crucified with Christ so that sin might lose its power in our lives. We are no longer slaves to sin. For when we died with Christ we were set free from the power of sin. And since we died with Christ, we know we will also live with him.
Romans 6:6-8

- How will your behavior and attitudes change as you move forward with a new (renewed) understanding of what God considers sexual sin. Be specific.

So submit to [the authority of] God. Resist the devil [stand firm against him] and he will flee from you.
James 4:7 AMP

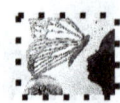

- Be honest: is submitting to God's authority a place of refuge or a place of restricted movement for you?

- Where are the places you know the devil continues to lurk around in your life? Think in terms of social influences and be specific.

12 Therefore let the one who thinks he stands firm [immune to temptation, being overconfident and self-righteous], take care that he does not fall [into sin and condemnation]. 13 No temptation [regardless of its source] has overtaken or enticed you that is not common to human experience [nor is any temptation unusual or beyond human resistance]; but God is faithful [to His word--He is compassionate and trustworthy], and He will not let you be tempted beyond your ability [to resist], but along with the temptation He [has in the past and is now and] will [always] provide the way out as well, so that you will be able to endure it [without yielding, and will overcome temptation with joy]. 14 Therefore, my beloved, run [keep far, far away] from [any sort of] idolatry [and that includes loving anything more than God, or participating in anything that leads to sin and enslaves the soul].
1 Corinthians 10:12-14 AMP

- On a separate piece of paper, name the idols of your past: people, places or things that took God's rightful place in your heart. Write them down and then tear the list up. You can bury it, burn it or simply throw it in the trash.

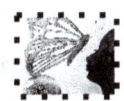

- Memorize Matthew 6:33. Put it up on your fridge, bathroom mirror and dash board. Make it one of your life verses to keep you straight.

33 "But seek first the kingdom of God and His righteousness, and all these things shall be added to you.
Matthew 6:33 NKJV

- Write out a three point pivot plan to flee in those times of temptation. Find a trusted friend and make them your accountability partner.

1.

2.

3.

Behold, I am doing a new thing; now it springs forth, do you not perceive it? I will make a way in the wilderness and rivers in the desert.
Isaiah 43:19 ESV

With eyes wide open, we must give the power of life and death back to God so that we can see the "new thing" He is doing in our lives. We can then begin to celebrate life from the "womb to the tomb" as "Whole Life" ambassadors of God. We can chart a new path forward giving Holy Spirit the reins to be our guide. As God's children, it is imperative that we govern ourselves according to what His original intent was:

- That life is precious from conception until natural death
- That sex should be reserved for marriage
- That marriage is a covenant relationship

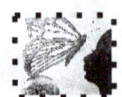

- That married households are the most stable environment for children to be raised in.
- That children are a unique and precious gift from God.

Outside of His plan lay the same shackles we have endeavored to remove these last eight weeks and dare I say, the last 300 years.

Acknowledging our past and all that we have been through both as a nation and as African American people, gives us a unique perspective on where we need to go now. We know that backwards is not forwards; not in this country. Nope. We have been released to walk forward in freedom; the shackles of conformity to what man says versus what God says about us have been completely removed. The Lord has graciously lifted us up out of the muck and mire and has set us free to live out our purpose for Him and Him alone.

We now know that a strong family unit is a spiritual force to be reckoned with! That means that any entity that works to weaken the family is, by definition, the enemy. We have God's permission to get excited again about His mandate to "be fruitful and multiply." As post-abortive women, we can go the extra mile to support the stressed and overwhelmed young men and women through their unexpected pregnancy. We can guide them past the snares of the enemy to help them see their child as a blessing and make an abortion "unthinkable." We can welcome our newest family members with the hopes and dreams we have been given by the Creator of the universe Himself; the same Creator who knew us before we were formed, knit us together in the womb, and had a purpose and a plan for our time here on earth. We can stand with our young folks by fulfilling our calling to walk beside them through the tough days of parenting. The Apostle Paul, in his letter to Titus graciously gave us the blueprint on how to help the youngins in Titus, chapter 2 verses 1-8:

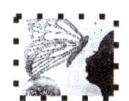

1 As for you, Titus, promote the kind of living that reflects wholesome teaching. 2 Teach the older men to exercise self-control, to be worthy of respect, and to live wisely. They must have sound faith and be filled with love and patience. 3 Similarly, teach the older women to live in a way that honors God. They must not slander others or be heavy drinkers. Instead, they should teach others what is good. 4 These older women must train the younger women to love their husbands and their children, 5 to live wisely and be pure, to work in their homes, to do good, and to be submissive to their husbands. Then they will not bring shame on the word of God. 6 In the same way, encourage the young men to live wisely. 7 And you yourself must be an example to them by doing good works of every kind. Let everything you do reflect the integrity and seriousness of your teaching. 8 Teach the truth so that your teaching can't be criticized. Then those who oppose us will be ashamed and have nothing bad to say about us.

Titus 2:1-8

Because of God's steadfast love, I have hope for our future. We now have the knowledge about our history that was crucial in understanding how we got stuck in the first place. With knowledge and wisdom we can be messengers of truth as we yield to God's will for our lives. The lives of our children will be testaments to the goodness of God and His hand in keeping us and prospering us despite all odds against us. We are no longer slaves to anyone but we have become joint heirs to the Kingdom promises of God right here in this land. And if He did it for you, He can do it for others. Let's shout, "Hallelujah" about that fact!!

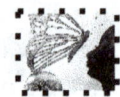

Check In:

Write out your plan to spend time daily with God. This should include practices such as:

- daily time in His Word
- prayer
- meditation on His Word
- memorizing bible verses
- singing hymns
- praising Him in dance
- journaling your prayers of gratitude.

Share your list with an accountability partner for support.

Expert Opinion: "Next" Steps

At Arise Daughter we have a saying: "Get ready, stay ready!" In order to help you do that, we offer one on one and small group mentoring sessions. Each meet up is designed to help you go to the next level and serve in the Kingdom of God in new ways. Be sure to schedule an appointment at: AriseDaughter@gmail.com.

- "Kingdom Marriage" by Tony Evans

Full Circle Moment of Reflection

Be still for a moment and reflect on what you have heard, read and experienced thus far. If God has given you a vision, write it down and place it deep in your heart.

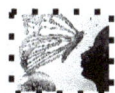

Write Your Prayer

Write a prayer of acknowledgement and gratitude for your new found freedom and for the ways God has moved in your life thus far. Thank Him in advance for what He is planning to do with the vision He gave to you.

Closing Songs and Celebration

- "Praise Party" by LeNasia Tyson.
- "Dancing in Freedom" "Gospel Dance Party Workout"
- "Blessings on Blessings" the B.O.B Bounce by Anthony Brown

Sis, you made it through!! To God be the glory for all that He has done these last few weeks, and all that He will continue to do in your life. Move forward with His direction and blessings, on to your "next" as you Arise, And Fly Free! Your sisters at Arise Daughter will continue to be with you in the days ahead. We want you to stay in touch so that we can continue to pray for you and fellowship with you.

One last assignment: If God has given you a vision about how you can contribute to the Kingdom, who you can share your healing with and how you can help others reconcile with Him then, trust it! He has chosen to reveal Himself to you and that is truly a gift! Pray for opportunities that align with God's will and share those with us at Arise Daughter. I will personally meet with you to help you strategize so that you can truly walk in freedom. Amen? Amen!

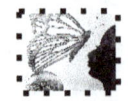

Epilogue

Let me acknowledge every person whose story was an inspiration to me. You are seen, you are valued and you are loved! For those who have yet to reveal their story, know that you are also seen, valued and loved by our heavenly Father. This book attempts the healing work that can only happen when Holy Spirit is in the midst doing what only He can do. There is clear recognition that for some, this journey has only taken its first baby steps. Many of us have other factors influencing our abortion trauma. Those factors may include multiple abortions; rape; molestation; incest; trafficking; coercion by a parent, friend, family member or medical professional; and issues of codependency that have now come to the surface because of the work of healing that you so courageously took on.

We encourage you to not look away from the broken places even if an emotional trigger rises up again. We also encourage you to remember that there is no condemnation that the enemy of your soul can throw up in your face! Romans 8:1 NKJV says it all: *[There is] therefore now no condemnation to those who are in Christ Jesus, who do not walk according to the flesh, but according to the Spirit.*

God wants your complete healing and He will not forsake you in what we believe are the "next" steps of your healing journey. Please go to: AriseArtists.com; SRTservices.org; H3Helpline.org; and SupportAfterAbortion.com for help in finding the necessary resources as you press on. And know that your healing community at Arise Daughter is here for you and would like to continue to walk with you every step of the way! Please contact us at: AriseDaughter@gmail.com to schedule a follow-up visit.

Amen and God bless as you "Arise, and Fly Free" and may God get the glory for it all!

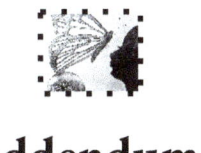

Addendum

Abortion Proofing Our Children

"Attend me, Virtue, thro' my youthful years! O leave me not to the false joys of time!"
'On Virtue' by Phillis Wheatley

I want to "abortion-proof" our children. It's a bold statement I know but I've come to realize that the evil laws of man will continue to corrupt minds if we don't touch hearts. I want the message to go out from trusted adults and authorities that abortion is wrong and that it will lead to destruction on multiple levels. I don't even want our kids to know where to obtain an abortion. And I want them to have the courage to speak out against the culture of death when they are challenged by pro-abortion peers. I don't want abortion facilities in our neighborhood where paid predators feel emboldened to call our sons and daughters off the streets to slaughter our babies. Our children need to know, before they are pressured into another opinion, that abortion goes against God's design for their lives. And the only way they will hear ANY of this is if we, the responsible adults, speak up and speak out while they are young!

Our culture of oversexualizing women and men has corrupted not only men's views of women but also our view of ourselves. In attempting to own who we are, many of us forget WHOSE we are and that we have been bought with a heavy price (1 Corinthians 6:20; 1 Corinthians 7:23). Our bodies are the temple of Holy Spirit (1 Corinthians 6:19) and are to be presented as a living sacrifice to God (Romans 12:1). Oh, how I wish someone had instilled these values in me!

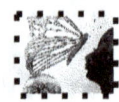

Virtue, chastity, and abstinence until marriage aren't even on most Americans' radar, but it will be up to us - those who have made different choices and suffered because of them - to help women and men of child-bearing age and younger to see their inherent worth, beauty and moral strength. Virginity isn't a small possession; it is of great wealth and to be protected.

If a man seduces a virgin who is not engaged to anyone and has sex with her, he must pay the customary bride price and marry her.
Exodus 22:16

Restore to me the joy of Your salvation, And sustain me with a willing spirit. Then I will teach transgressors Your ways, And sinners shall be converted and return to You.
Psalm 51:12-13 AMP

Potential Strategies to Abortion Proof Our Children
(This is a starter and not meant to be exhaustive.)

1. Have conversations about purity of body, mind and spirit. Use [this Facebook post](https://www.facebook.com/share/r/XxTnPqirSFzrqQ1t/?mibextid=xfxF2i) by Brian Jones Jr. as a starter for the conversation
https://www.facebook.com/share/r/XxTnPqirSFzrqQ1t/?mibextid=xfxF2i
    - The book of Proverbs was written to help parents have those conversations. Check out the books:
      - [Proverbs: A Strong Man Is Wise](#) by Vince Miller
      - [A Devotional Journey Through Proverbs: 31 Reflections and Insights](#) by Our Daily Bread.

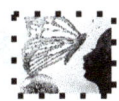

- Also view the Facebook post explaining "Why Christ is Lord of Our Bodies".

2. Encourage your church youth leadership to offer Christian dating discussions. What does healthy dating look like and what does sex outside of marriage mean to God?

3. Discuss the difference between saying you are a Christian and acting like you are a Christian.
   Here is a Facebook clip on spiritual integrity.

4. Offer a class on baby development - something not adequately taught in schools. Bring in the science *and* the theology so that young people make the appropriate connections using baby models, colorful illustrations, videos and bible verses that speak to life before and in the womb. Show the "Baby Olivia" video at home and marvel together at the majesty of life. Show the First trimester baby models of development so that the "blob of tissue" and "clump of cells" lie doesn't stick.

5. Be brave. Show your children the different types of abortion and what happens to the baby and the mom. Use the website: www.abortionprocedures.com for detailed facts about pill and surgical abortions so that no one can lie to them about what an abortion is. Go to the YouTube stream: The Procedure for an animated enactment of an abortion story. Every 13 year old already knows that killing babies is wrong; this will reinforce their convictions. Watch with them, answer questions, have tissues ready and cry together.

6. Watch this video, Oxytocin: The Big Deal About Sex that describes the chemical bonds created during sex. Discuss that, from a biblical (God's) standpoint, sex=marriage.

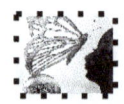

7. Discuss *date rape*, what it is and what it looks like for both boys and girls. Talk about having an escape plan BEFORE the situation heats up and that kissing can be interpreted as "yes" to sex for many young men.

8. Teach our children what *spiritual warfare* means, how to recognize a spiritual issue, how Holy Spirit prompts us to pay attention and the weapons needed to fight effectively.
    - Dr. Cindy Trimm's book: The Art of War for Spiritual Battle
    - Facebook video on Spiritual Warfare and Forgiveness

9. Encourage and model sensitivity to and participation in the social justice issues that continue to plague African Americans. Issues such as:
    - Lack of adequate prenatal care providers in high density population areas.
    - Diverting funding of abortion to funding emergency child care centers and maternal homes.
    - Zoning that includes adequate lower income housing options in cities.
    - Addressing the normalizing of low literacy in city schools.
    - Pressing for a curriculum that includes fetal development, parenting skills and other basic life skills.
    - Education on sexual grooming - what it looks like from the predator's viewpoint and how to counteract it.
    - Understanding societal injustices towards African Americans and the stressors that accompany *being black*. (5 minute video with Dr. Joy Degruy)
    - Advocating for 6 months paid parental leave and subsidized child care.

10. Continue the college campus awareness and activism started by Pro-Black, Pro-Life to champion Whole Life issues and counter the Planned Parenthood narrative. The college environment is

where your work as a parent can be undone. Stay in touch with your child and what is influencing them. Connect them with a community like Campus Crusade for Christ, or Christian Athletes so that they have a trusted tribe.

11. Listen to men and their abortion stories for another perspective. After all, men are a vital part of the equation; their voice and influence matters:
    A. "Overtime with Damien: Life After Abortion: A Man's Perspective with Anthony Hayes"
    B. "Why Men Are Also Responsible for Abortion"

12. Start an AND Campaign chapter in your city hosted by your church and train to become an AND Campaign Ambassador.

13. Be prepared to have the, "You are already having sex, now what?" talk. Play this YouTube video: "The Wait: Why We Regret Having Sex Before Marriage" Discuss the ABSOLUTE necessity for gynecological checkups for both sexes as soon as you suspect sexual activity has occurred. Teens hardly ever consider pregnancy as the outcome of sex but sexually transmitted infections almost NEVER enter their minds.

14. Help your children include godly music into their lives and playlists. Joy FM (modern Christian)/ LF Radio (Christian Rap) are stations that appeal to teens and are relevant to Christ-centered living.

15. Download the YouVersion app on their phone and find a daily devotion that you can do together.

References

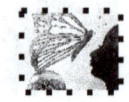

Bible References:
1. Blue Letter Bible, https://www.blueletterbible.org/
2. Bible.com, https://bible.com/bible/116/exo.22.16.NLT
3. Our Daily Bread Publishing, https://ourdailybreadpublishing.org/a-devotional-journey-through-proverbs.html
4. YouVersion Bible, https://www.youversion.com/

Prologue
1. Sexually Related Trauma Services, https://srtservices.org/
2. Arise Daughter, "Jackson, Mississippi Testimony," YouTube video, Sylvia Blakely, April 17, 2022, https://www.youtube.com/watch?v=5-hL4U-hAY4
3. AND (&) Campaign, https://andcampaign.org/
4. Arise Daughter, "Whole Life Project," YouTube video, June 1, 2023, https://www.youtube.com/watch?v=fDxgMvN75UY
5. Sylvia Blakely, "Silent No More" Campaign Testimony, YouTube video, Washington D.C., January 21, 2022, https://www.youtube.com/watch?v=yb8UGEUdgp4
6. Sylvia Blakely, "Decades", YouTube video, June 12, 2021, https://www.youtube.com/watch?v=-qCaetlTKR4
7. Pro Black, Pro Life, https://problackprolife.com/
8. Live Action, "I Regret My Abortion - Sylvia's Story: Can't Stay Silent" Testimony, YouTube video, Sylvia Blakely, September 28, 2022, https://www.youtube.com/watch?v=7olCOabFJrE
9. Lisa Rowe, *Support After Abortion: A Catalyst for Change with Sylvia Blakely*, Spotify interview in the Support After Abortion podcast, March 2021, https://open.spotify.com/episode/71aoKDxu9fVCHPLWGKJuDU?si=09385f68cc5f4212&nd=1&dlsi=7c18b4171d874461
10. Arise Daughter YouTube Channel, https://www.youtube.com/channel/UCSLQp91fsfSfpgbqlVqlW6A

11. [Tony Evans: The Urban Alternative, https://tonyevans.org/](https://tonyevans.org/)
12. [Pray.com,](https://www.pray.com/) https://www.pray.com/
13. Joe Carter, ["How to Keep A Spiritual Journal"](https://www.thegospelcoalition.org/course/journaling/#course-introduction), The Gospel Coalition, https://www.thegospelcoalition.org/course/journaling/#course-introduction
14. [Free Faith Coloring Page for Adults to Give You Joy](https://thecreatorsclassroom.com/free-coloring-pages-for-adults-to-bring-joy-to-your-life/), https://thecreatorsclassroom.com/free-coloring-pages-for-adults-to-bring-joy-to-your-life/
15. Self Love Rainbow, ["Your Boundaries Matter"](https://www.instagram.com/p/Cn9qkD5uOVh/), Instagram post, https://www.instagram.com/p/Cn9qkD5uOVh/
16. Channel Kayy, ["Effective Ways To Say, 'No'"](https://www.tiktok.com/t/ZT8pWjG31/), TikTok video, https://www.tiktok.com/t/ZT8pWjG31/
17. Sylvia Blakely, [Virtual Wellness Basket](https://www.canva.com/design/DAF8hhdlxWU/BV0AtSVKy6YenB73DvudfQ/view?utm_content=DAF8hhdlxWU&utm_campaign=designshare&utm_medium=link&utm_source=editor), Canva creation, March 2024, https://www.canva.com/design/DAF8hhdlxWU/BV0AtSVKy6YenB73DvudfQ/view?utm_content=DAF8hhdlxWU&utm_campaign=designshare&utm_medium=link&utm_source=editor
18. CeCe Winans, ["Believe For It"](https://www.youtube.com/watch?v=n4ggKHAK_xk), YouTube video, February 12, 2021, https://www.youtube.com/watch?v=n4ggKHAK_xk
19. Todd Galberth, ["It's Your Breath"](https://www.youtube.com/watch?v=KXxBkcZTF0c), YouTube video, November 15, 2021, https://www.youtube.com/watch?v=KXxBkcZTF0c

Chapter 1: Understanding Our Unique History
1. Sojourner Truth, ["Ain't I A Woman"](https://etc.usf.edu/lit2go/185/civil-rights-and-conflict-in-the-united-states-selected-speeches/3089/aint-i-a-woman/), 1851, https://etc.usf.edu/lit2go/185/civil-rights-and-conflict-in-the-united-states-selected-speeches/3089/aint-i-a-woman/
2. Harriet Jacobs, *Incidents in the Life of a Slave Girl*; 1861, (Available for free on Google Books and Librivox Audiobooks.)
3. Frederick Douglass, *Narrative of the Life of Fredrick Douglass,* 1845, (Available for free on Google books and Librivox Audiobooks.)
4. Solomon Northup, *12 Years A Slave*, *1853*

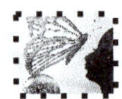

5. "Sexual Exploitation of the Enslaved", https://encyclopediavirginia.org/entries/sexual-exploitation-of-the-enslaved/
6. Richard C. Francis, *Epigenetics: How Environment Shapes Our Genes*, 2012
7. Ida B. Wells, *The Red Record*, 1895
8. Ida B. Wells, *On Lynchings*, 1892
9. Isabel Wilkerson, *The Warmth of Other Suns*, October 2011
10. Isabel Wilkerson, *Caste: The Origins of Our Discontent*, August 2020
11. Dorothy Roberts, *Killing The Black Body*, December 1998
12. Title X Program Funding History, https://opa.hhs.gov/grant-programs/archive/title-x-program-archive/title-x-program-funding-history
13. *Maafa 21: Black Genocide in 21st Century America*, directed and produced by Mark Crutcher, 2009
14. Bible Project, "Character of God" video, YouTube. https://youtu.be/nxwzq1PJlmM?si=V-us3ycBEzkZO7C0
15. FaithfullyPlanted.com, "How to Pray The Lord's Prayer" https://faithfullyplanted.com/lords-prayer-personal-guide/
16. Peter Collins, "I Don't Feel Noways Tired", YouTube video, August 23, 2020, https://www.youtube.com/watch?v=NQj1ZfSJpEg
17. Reverend James Cleveland, "I Don't Feel Noways Tired", YouTube video, Recorded 1978, https://www.youtube.com/watch?v=_Cw75v2uqts
18. Anthony Brown, "Deep Enough", YouTube video, March 23, 2017, https://youtu.be/rwLslsnahb4?si=rfjBuvrd7VpwdKAt
19. Maverick City Music, "Breathe", YouTube video, February 11, 2022 https://www.youtube.com/watch?v=mR-D3bvi-4E&pp=ygUVYnJlYXRoZSBtYXZlcmljayBjaXR5

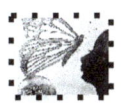

20. *New Life Ministries*, "Feelings Journey", https://us17.campaign-archive.com/?e=93552b7d04&u=d68cfe6f434a19c695f9f8b24&id=c164e366b3

Chapter 2: Acknowledging Our "Choice(s)" and the Forces Behind Them

1. Booker T. Washington, https://www.history.com/topics/black-history/booker-t-washington
2. Ibram X. Kendi, "Learning for Justice", TeachingTolerance.org : a project of the Southern Poverty Law Center.
3. Jeffrey Pokorak, "Rape as a Badge of Slavery: The Legal Histoy of, and Remedies for, Prosecutorial Race-of-Victim Charging Disparities, September 2006, *Nevada Law Journal*: Vol. 7: Iss. 1, Article 2. https://scholars.law.unlv.edu/nlj/vol7/iss1/2/
4. Alana Semuels: 'I Don't Have Faith in Doctors Anymore'. Women Say They Were Pressured Into Long Term Birth Control. May 13 2024 Time Magazine https://time.com/6976918/long-term-birth-control-reproductive-coercion/
5. GotQuestions.org, "Spiritual Strongholds"
6. Headfulness, "Box Breathing for Stress: 4x4" for Stress, YouTube video, December 6, 2023, https://www.youtube.com/shorts/Pu38MLUgzZs
7. California Institute of Integral Studies, *Revisiting Joy DeGruy: Post-Traumatic Slave Syndrome*, YouTube video, January 19, 2018, https://www.youtube.com/watch?v=0ZNwZAWl-WE
8. AJ+, *Post Traumatic Slave Syndroome. How is it Different from PTSD?* YouTube video, Joy DeGruy, November 9, 2019, https://www.youtube.com/watch?v=Rorgjdvphek
9. Dharius Daniels, "Strangling Strongholds" YouTube video, September 24, 2024, https://www.youtube.com/live/J3SVggeyvag?si=0W0gYu5LEipjqddJ
10. Timeline Example, https://www.ncbar.org/wp-content/uploads/2022/02/Timeline-Visual.png

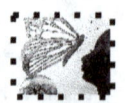

11. Fred Hammond, "Draw Nigh (Psalm 42:1)", YouTube video, Recorded 1996, https://www.youtube.com/watch?v=A3US86Zm0jU

Chapter 3: Recognizing Our Wounds

1. Joy DeGruy, "Post Traumatic Slave Syndrome", www.joydegruy.com
2. Michelle Alexander, *The New Jim Crow*, January 16, 2012, https://newjimcrow.com/about/buy
3. H3Helpline, https://h3helpline.org/
4. Amanda D'Ambrosio, "Study: Relief Most Common Emotion 5 Years Post-Abortion", January 13, 2020, https://www.medpagetoday.com/obgyn/pregnancy/84345
5. David Reardon, "The Abortion and Mental Health Controversy," October 29, 2018, https://www.ncbi.nlm.nih.gov/pmc/articles/PMC6207970/
6. "Oxytocin: the Big Deal About Sex", YouTube video April 10, 2021. https://youtu.be/tUBlQABIs10?si=Souh77c-9guG9cTi
7. "First Trimester Baby Models"
8. Live Action, Baby Olivia, https://babyolivia.liveaction.org/share/
9. Gentle Birthing Video, Facebook video, https://www.facebook.com/reel/600613595377596
10. Operation Outcry, https://www.operationoutcry.org/
11. Allina Health, "Head-to-Toe Relaxation", YouTube video, October 24, 2016, https://www.youtube.com/watch?v=A1z4Nq_N2do
12. Spirit of Humanity Forum, Dr. Joy DeGruy About Resolving Trauma and How We Can All Be the Healing", April 5, 2021, https://www.youtube.com/watch?v=X9KfhemgUf4
13. Voddie Baucham "Brokenness," YouTube video August 11, 2013, https://youtu.be/GVow8rSQwiA?si=ADY_0GfNm1liqleR
14. Sylvia Blakely, "Now and Later" Healing Exercise, Canva

15. Fred Hammond, "Prodigal Son (Psalm 32:5)," YouTube video, Recorded 1996, https://www.youtube.com/watch?v=Ztb8QM2TtWE
16. Donald Lawrence, "Deliver Me (This Is My Exodus)," YouTube video, Recorded 2017, https://www.youtube.com/watch?v=KwYJv455Zmk
17. Sylvia Blakely, *Moral Injury Through a Biblical Lens*, February 13, 2022, https://arisedaughter.wixsite.com/website/post/moral-injury-through-a-biblical-lens
18. Sylvia Blakely, Part 2: Moral Injury Through a Biblical Lens, March 7, 2022, https://arisedaughter.wixsite.com/website/post/part-2-moral-injury-through-a-biblical-lens
19. Sylvia Blakely, Part 3: Moral Injury Through a Biblical Lens, March 8, 2022, https://arisedaughter.wixsite.com/website/post/part-3-moral-injury-through-a-biblical-lens
20. Arise Daughter Wellness Basket on Canva https://www.canva.com/design/DAF8hhdlxWU/BV0AtSVKy6YenB73DvudfQ/view?utm_content=DAF8hhdlxWU&utm_campaign=designshare&utm_medium=link&utm_source=editor

Chapter 4: Understanding Our Pain

1. *Zora Neale Hurston: Claiming a Space,* PBS, Directed by Tracy Heather Strain, produced by Randall MacLowry and executive produced by Cameo George, January 17, 2023, https://www.pbs.org/wgbh/americanexperience/films/zora-neale-hurston-claiming-space/#part01
2. The National Institute of Health: "The Facts and Doubts About the Beginning of Life and Personality" https://www.ncbi.nlm.nih.gov/pmc/articles/PMC7245522/#:~:text=The%20biological%20line%20of%20existence,male%20and%20female%20reproductive%20tracts.
3. Syracuse University, "The Moral Injury Project: What Is Moral Injury", https://moralinjuryproject.syr.edu/about-moral-injury/

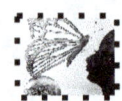

4. Live Action, "I Regret My Abortion - Sylvia's Story: Can't Stay Silent", YouTube video, Sylvia Blakely, September 28, 2022, https://www.youtube.com/watch?v=7olCOabFJrE
5. Freda Abbott-Ayodele: "The Mask Exercise", 2024
6. Fred Hammond, "Breathe Into Me Oh Lord (Psalm 119:26)", YouTube video, Recorded 1996, https://www.youtube.com/watch?v=rVVgDuwrcXI
7. Tonex, "Lord, Make Me Over", YouTube video, Recorded 2004, https://www.youtube.com/watch?v=9t60fl39Iy8
8. Fred Hammond and United Tenors, "I'm In The Midst Of It All", YouTube video, Recorded 2013, https://www.youtube.com/watch?v=JE7lQBzPrkc
9. Isaac Carree, "In The Middle", YouTube video, Recorded 2011, https://www.youtube.com/watch?v=uxtdql1Crsc

Chapter 5: Dealing With the Anger

1. Dr. Maya Angelou quote on anger.
2. Mayo Clinic: "Chronic Stress Puts Your Health At Risk"
3. Kim Pratt, "Psychology Tools: What is Anger? A Secondary Emotion", Healthy Psych, February 3, 2014, https://healthypsych.com/psychology-tools-what-is-anger-a-secondary-emotion/#google_vignette
4. Roxanne Fields: "The Iceberg Exercise"
5. NF, "Happy", YouTube video, Premiered April 7, 2023. https://youtu.be/jDjF7BtJazk?si=slVuc0e_JEB8qG1t
6. Lamont Sanders, "He Kept Me", YouTube video, Recorded 2020, https://www.youtube.com/watch?v=tuXNWQLdJsY

Chapter 6: Grieving Our Losses

1. Beloved, directed by Jonathan Demme, 1998
2. Dr. Martin Luther King Jr., Why We Can't Wait, 1964
3. E. Joanne Angelo, "Portraits of Grief in the Aftermath of Abortion", Hope After Abortion,

https://hopeafterabortion.com/?p=106&gclid=Cj0KCQiA6fafBhC1ARIsAIJjL8kL0Y-xqilwUV9GlsVXDdvjbbXGF7KzaayvrsrUon9lti1qbBm3xjAaAh5cEALw_wcB

4. Koryn Hawthorne, "Cry", June 2, 2023.
https://youtu.be/OXRbvGEmlMc?si=3pggmO5fwexnvXxD
5. Rev. Dr. LaRuth, "Encouragement For Those Who Suffer In Silence". https://www.amazon.com/Encouragement-Those-Who-Suffer-Silence/dp/B0CYKHGD1V
6. Litsa Williams, "Grief After Abortion: Healing From Unspoken Loss", What's Your Grief, https://whatsyourgrief.com/grief-abortion-healing-unspoken-loss/
7. The Book of Lamentations by the Bible Project https://youtu.be/p8GDFPdaQZQ?si=uxUlq3kELYvBl1e5
8. "Made In the Image Of God", We Are Messengers, September 11, 2020, https://www.youtube.com/watch?v=8yV0pu60Uqs

Chapter 7: Forgiving the Unforgivable

1. Maya Angelou: NPR interview
https://www.npr.org/2013/03/31/175493858/in-a-new-memoir-maya-angelou-recalls-how-a-lady-became-mom
2. The Bible Project, "God's Consistent Posture Toward All Humanity," YouTube video, September 22, 2020, https://www.youtube.com/watch?v=ABPVVw_aw44
3. Therapist Aid, "How to do Progressive Muscle Relaxation", YouTube video, August 3, 2014, https://www.youtube.com/watch?v=1nZEdqcGVzo
4. Sylvia Blakely, Wellness Basket, March 2024, https://www.canva.com/design/DAF8hhdlxWU/BV0AtSVKy6YenB73DvudfQ/view?utm_content=DAF8hhdlxWU&utm_campaign=designshare&utm_medium=link&utm_source=editor
5. Dr. Barbara L. Peacock: "Soul Care for Today's Woman"
https://youtu.be/OCSURaKD3pc?si=QZz5lc4qSCKszJuW

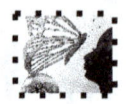

6. Dr. Voddie Baucham: "Forgiveness" https://youtu.be/YdmG87-skWw?si=IrgbKC8elQRjm-19
7. Forgiveness: Extend an act of kindness, Priscilla Shirer on Better Together September 12, 2023.
https://youtu.be/ndhePFgRTao?si=am6guRv5dAPWhS5A
8. Oprah Daily, "Tyler Perry Tells Oprah How He Was Able to Forgive His Father", YouTube video, February 6, 2024, https://www.youtube.com/watch?v=x30lErGONUQ
9. Tasha Page-Lockhart and Bryan Popin, "Beautiful Savior (feat. Bryan Popin)", YouTube Video, Recorded 2017, https://www.youtube.com/watch?v=4v-KRMAYbwc
10. Brian Courtney Wilson, "A Great Work (Sirius XM Performance)", YouTube Video, Recorded 2018, https://www.youtube.com/watch?v=0ZRMqToyPss

Chapter 8: Restoring Hope

1. Langston Hughes: "Mother to Son" The Poetry Foundation.
2. Inside FBCG, "I Am Who God Says I Am", Priscilla Shirer, YouTube video, October 13, 2023, https://www.youtube.com/watch?v=CF0DsSm_5ko
3. Young Scot, "Box Breathing Technique", YouTube video, October 20, 2022, https://www.youtube.com/shorts/5WUsrJawuIg
4. Gospel Music Unlimited, "For My Good", Todd Galberth, YouTube video, 2019, https://youtu.be/qml34EOFU_w
5. "Worth Fighting For", Brian Courtney Wilson, YouTube video, 2014, https://www.youtube.com/watch?v=EojzHQqApKM
6. "Sea of Forgetfulness", Helen Baylor, YouTube video, 2011 https://youtu.be/1o542-0NcJQ?si=wt98uUQZ1pvIgfQU

Chapter 9: Walking In Freedom

1. "Oxytocin, the Big Deal About Sex", YouTube Video, Radical Relationships.

2. Tony Evans, "Kingdom Marriage", YouTube video, November 23, 2022, https://www.youtube.com/watch?v=23yC-rWsOpA

3. "Praise Party", LeNasia Tyson, YouTube video, July 13, 2018, https://www.youtube.com/watch?v=tFDEmNSpViQ
4. "Gospel Dance Party Workout" YouTube video by Grow With Jo, June 10, 2021,https://youtu.be/nLJhTkLhK5U?si=8FQnwD4oGBhmUxT0
5. "Blessings on Blessings" BOB Bounce, Anthony Brown, July 19, 2019, https://youtu.be/nLJhTkLhK5U?si=8FQnwD4oGBhmUxT0

Addendum
1. *A Devotional Journey Through Proverbs: 31 Reflections and Insights from Our Daily Bread,* Our Daily Bread Publishing, March 1, 2021 https://ourdailybreadpublishing.org/a-devotional-journey-through-proverbs.html
2. Priscilla Shirer, ",
3. *Proverbs: A Strong Man Is Wise A 30-Day Devotional,* Be Resolute, https://beresolute.org/product/proverbs-a-strong-man-is-wise/
4. Baby Olivia development video by LiveAction
5. First Trimester Baby Models
6. Oxytocin: The Big Deal About Sex by Radical Relationships
7. *The Art of War by Dr.* Cindy Trimm,, August 3, 2010, https://www.amazon.com/Art-War-Spiritual-Battle-Strategies/dp/1599798727
8. AJ+, "Post Traumatic Slave Syndrome. How is it Different from PTSD?", Joy DeGruy, YouTube video, November 8, 2019, https://youtu.be/Rorgjdvphek?si=VyzQChmJDcDn2h-s
9. Pro-Black Pro-Life, Cherilynn Holloway, https://problackprolife.com/
10. Damien and Kenady Nash, Overtime with Damien, "Life After Abortion: A Man's Perspective with Anthony Hayes. YouTube

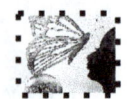

Video, September 9, 2020, https://youtu.be/NvFcQmTsvqM?si=wwtd23ymEx3CTWzo
11. AND Campaign, https://andcampaign.org/
12. The Makhs, The Wait: Why We Regret Having Sex Before Marriage. YouTube, July 11, 2021, https://youtu.be/H_d-t7IOG_M?si=0g1PO3KYk7Fj8Ffk
13. Ascension Presents, "Why Men Are Also Responsible for Abortion", YouTube video, January 14, 2020, https://www.youtube.com/watch?v=qijSoXet56U

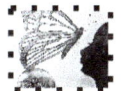

Arise Daughter Offers Mentoring

There is so much waiting for you on the other side of this healing journey: so much more! Your sisters at Arise Daughter are ready to help you explore your "next"; whether it is a place to share your testimony, another healing study or an opportunity to help another sister out of the muck and mire. We would love to walk beside you as you explore your options.

You can find us at:
AriseDaughter.org and AriseArtists.com.
@arisedaughterfl on Facebook & Instagram
@arisedaughter3 on TikTok
Arise Daughter on YouTube
Our Spotify Channel is: Arise Daughter

Join our Memorial Garden Movement to honor your child(ren).

NOTES:

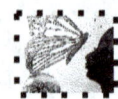

Comments about, "Arise, And Fly Free":

- "SO WELL DONE! I am deeply thrilled for this e-book to come out, how God will use it, and the impact it will have on so many! Amanda.Forgiven@gmail.com. Click to see Amanda's testimony.

- "I had no idea, and I'm almost ashamed that I didn't know!!!!!! My mouth is still open. I read the excerpt in doses, and I've included some notes I took while pondering the wealth of information and the background of the blatant, pre-meditated system of black genocide. This is critical knowledge that should be required reading for all African-American teenagers." Sharon

This curriculum is dedicated to the women of African descent who have been targeted by the abortion industry and succumbed to their rhetoric. It has been written with love and with you in mind. May God get the glory for the healing that only He can provide! Sylvia Blakely.

About the author: Sylvia Blakely is a post-abortive woman passionate about helping other women heal and walk in freedom. She is a devoted daughter of the Most High God, a wife of 36 years and an aunt and godmother. She founded Arise Daughter and Arise Artists ministries after her own healing journey began in 2020, almost 40 years after her abortion. To hear her testimony, go to: Sylvia Blakely LiveAction

www.ingramcontent.com/pod-product-compliance
Lightning Source LLC
Chambersburg PA
CBHW080343170426
43194CB00014B/2672